RUNES
– for the –
Green Witch

"Nicolette Miele's *Runes for the Green Witch* is a masterclass in correspondences, providing a unique and holistic approach to the intersection of runic mysteries and herbalism. Prepare to be guided by Nicolette's passion and expertise; from the introduction to the runic formulary of oils, teas, spell bottles, and more, you'll fall in love with the system presented in this book. Filled with folklore, medicinal applications, personal insight, and clever correspondences, *Runes for the Green Witch* is sure to become a classic reference book for the ages."

NICHOLAS PEARSON, AUTHOR OF
FLOWER ESSENCES FROM THE WITCH'S GARDEN
AND *STONES OF THE GODDESS*

"This book is like having four volumes wrapped up in one. Not only is there well-researched information on the runes themselves, the book also offers correspondences for each of the Futhark to use for magical purposes. This comprehensive herbal grimoire knits plant magic into the fold, and the reader is also presented with personal experiential tales offered by the author."

MAJA D'AOUST, WITCH OF THE DAWN AND
AUTHOR OF *FAMILIARS IN WITCHCRAFT*

RUNES
– for the –
Green Witch

AN HERBAL
GRIMOIRE

A Sacred Planet Book

Nicolette Miele

Destiny Books
Rochester, Vermont

Destiny Books
One Park Street
Rochester, Vermont 05767
www.DestinyBooks.com

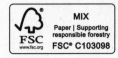

Destiny Books is a division of Inner Traditions International

Sacred Planet Books are curated by Richard Grossinger, Inner Traditions editorial board member and cofounder and former publisher of North Atlantic Books. The Sacred Planet collection, published under the umbrella of the Inner Traditions family of imprints, includes works on the themes of consciousness, cosmology, alternative medicine, dreams, climate, permaculture, alchemy, shamanic studies, oracles, astrology, crystals, hyperobjects, locutions, and subtle bodies.

The information within this book is in no way intended to diagnose, treat, cure, prevent any disease, or replace professional medical advice. Never ingest or administer herbal remedies without first performing the necessary thorough research and assessment of the possible risks. Neither the author nor the publisher is responsible for any mishandlings that result from the following information of *Runes for the Green Witch*. Always practice safe magick.

Cataloging-in-Publication Data for this title is available from the Library of Congress

ISBN 978-1-64411-866-5 (print)
ISBN 978-1-64411-867-2 (ebook)

Printed and bound in the United States by Lake Book Manufacturing, LLC

10 9 8 7 6 5 4 3 2 1

Text design and layout by Virginia Scott Bowman
This book was typeset in Garamond Premier Pro and Gill Sans with Geographica Hand and Bradley DJR used as display typefaces

To send correspondence to the author of this book, mail a first-class letter to the author c/o Inner Traditions • Bear & Company, One Park Street, Rochester, VT 05767, and we will forward the communication, or contact the author directly at **handfulsofdust.com**.

Scan the QR code and save 25% at InnerTraditions.com. Browse over 2,000 titles on spirituality, the occult, ancient mysteries, new science, holistic health, and natural medicine.

This book is dedicated to my grandfather, Mark,

and

to the loving memory of my nanas,
Gloria and Donna.

ACKNOWLEDGMENTS

Special thanks to everyone at Inner Traditions, Richard Grossinger, Eric Benson, Sus Kushner-Benson, Dad, Kate Moran, Sean Möwer, J. J. Miele, Jaquan Smith, Larry Brooks, Lena Wilde, Judy Ann Nock, Michelle Stuart, Caelynn Hartwig, Amanda Ruth, Beth Songer, Omie, Lunar, Sabbath, Indie, and my son, Maddox—the coolest person I know.

CONTENTS

The First Aett

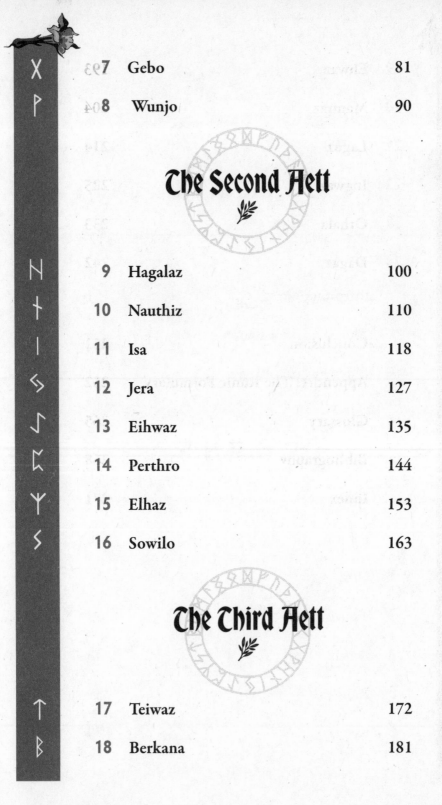

General Safety and Wildcrafting Guidelines

Wildcrafting: The proper identification of a plant is crucial and can save lives. Plants have doppelgangers—for example, the benign wild carrot plant, which is also known as Queen Anne's lace, is nearly identical to poison hemlock, which can be fatal if ingested. The only slight difference between the two plants is the appearance of their stems. Field guides are particularly valuable for foraging, and you can find ones specific to your region of the globe. Plant identification apps are also available via smart phones. For the safety and respect of our ecosystems and the Earth as a whole, please be informed on which plants are overharvested (or worse, endangered) before collecting. When you do forage, it is best to clip the stalks rather than remove the entire root; that way the plant may replenish itself.

Essential oils: The essential oils of plants are best suited for external use and should be diluted with carrier oils. Ingesting essential oils is not recommended, as it can do more harm than good. Always check the safety guidelines of an oil before use—especially if you are pregnant, breastfeeding, or coping with a physical illness of any kind.

INTRODUCTION

And into the forest I go to lose my mind and find my soul.

JOHN MUIR

Real magick and witchcraft are not what we see in movies and television. Real witches cannot snap their fingers to smite an enemy (unfortunately), nor can they mount a broom and fly through the night skies (also very unfortunate). There are many ways to define what magick and witchcraft really are, and the definitions may even differ from person to person. Occultist Aleister Crowley defined *magick* as "the science and art of causing change to occur in conformity with will."[*] Author Christopher Penczak wrote "Witchcraft is the building of sacred space, in myself, in my life, in my environment."[†] I agree with both statements and raise them a "Witchcraft is the process of actively seeking answers to the mysteries and working forces behind existence itself"—or something like that. One might argue that my definition suggests scientific inquiry, and I'd argue that witchcraft is a mechanism for exploring not-yet-understood natural phenomena.

The truth is, there's nothing *super*natural about magick—it's just as natural as the sun, the trees, and the processes of birth and death. Before humanity understood the tides, the seasons, and the phases of the moon, we applied supernatural explanations to such processes, which birthed many of the goddesses and gods we still work with

---

[*]Aleister Crowley, *Magick, Liber ABA, Book 4* (York Beach, Maine: Weiser Books, 1994), 128.

[†]Christopher Penczak, *The Inner Temple of Witchcraft: Magick, Meditation, and Psychic Development* (Woodbury, Minn.: Llewellyn Publications, 2003), 3.

today. Today we understand the science behind such things and no longer label them as supernatural. Simply put, magick is natural phenomena we are not yet able to grasp. Regardless, it is practiced by many who are trying like hell to grasp or even glimpse such things.

When it comes to the meaning of magick, my mind rewinds back to something I heard in the Incubus song "New Skin" when I was a teen. It's a quote by architect and philosopher Buckminster Fuller and states, "Up to the twentieth century, reality was everything humans could touch, smell, see, and hear. Since the initial publication of the chart of the electromagnetic spectrum, humans have learned that what they can touch, smell, see, and hear is less than one-millionth of reality." *Less than one-millionth of reality. One-millionth!* I think it's safe to say that the first time I heard that, my mind exploded all over the damn place, and honestly, it still explodes to this day just thinking about it. There is so much more to the world, to the cosmos, than we can ever know—much of it going on right in front of our faces, which can be a fascinating yet frustrating notion. Buckminster Fuller's quote alone launched me on a full-scale quest to search out the parts of reality we cannot readily sense; that and Plato's Allegory of the Cave, which in my opinion portrays an idea similar to that of the quote. This quest inevitably led me on a fast-track to practicing magick, and I haven't slowed since.

It's an interesting time to be a witch. We no longer have to wonder how we're to learn our crafts, and even better, we no longer have to worry about being burned at the stake, although I'm sure there are still some cranky folks out there who wouldn't mind making examples of us! *Sucks to be them.* Another perk for us modern practitioners is that we have at our disposal an impressive array of trade tools to aid us in spell work and ritual. We are fortunate to live in a time where there's no shortage of local and online metaphysical shops, the likes of which would surely astound our magickal predecessors. With the internet at our fingertips, these tools of the trade are no longer limited by locality. One doesn't have to live in Africa to have easy access to frankincense or in northern Europe to get their hands on sources of runic knowledge and mysticism.

The markets of new age, spiritual, and occult offerings are raging these days. According to the World Economic Forum, "[Spirituality] annually contributes about $1.2 trillion dollars of socioeconomic value to the United States economy and shows no signs of slowing down."* There's some serious capitalism happening in spiritual communities today, which is inevitable given the rise in popularity, not to mention the witch's need to make money for survival.

Now, I'm not here to make anyone feel bad about how they spend their own money. Like my wonderful nanas before me, I am a shopping gal through and through. In my home I have my own private ritual room (or *witch cave* as my son calls it), which is filled floor to ceiling with occult books, runes, tarot decks, oracle decks, crystals, deity statues, apothecary jars filled with herbs and resins (too many jars!), and other random tools and knickknacks. Honestly, most days it looks like an occult shop blew up inside the tiny room, and I *love it*. Sometimes I have to remind myself, however, to cool it on the candle purchases or that I don't really need another tarot deck. While there will always be a part of me that fantasizes about giving away all my belongings and moving to a small, secluded cabin in the woods where I live off the land entirely, I'm also a realist, and I like my stuff. It's all about balance. Even moderation in moderation. I learned that last part from a fortune cookie.

The idea for this book came not only from my passion for rune work and herbcraft but also from my need to walk my talk and put nature back in the forefront of my practice. When it comes down to it, one only *really* needs intention, focus, and the ability to raise and direct energy; but for those of us (me!) who like to employ various spiritual tools, or *allies,* nature is always stocked with the best available; and what better way to return to our roots than through working with manifestations of the Earth and cosmos?

The following is a quick cautionary tale regarding magickal necessities. When I was eleven years old, I acquired my very first book of

*Brian J. Grim, "Religion May Be Bigger Business Than We Thought. Here's Why." World Economic Forum (website), January 5, 2017.

spells. Prior to this purchase my only knowledge of witchcraft was what I had seen in the 1996 movie *The Craft,* which is still one of my favorite movies to this day. I was completely mesmerized by Nancy and had firmly decided that when I grew up, I was going to be her—except for the whole murderous rage and insane asylum thing at the end. But I digress. At my young age I was not aware of focused intent and energy. I assumed that magick resided solely within the words, ingredients, tools, and actions of a ritual—the incantations, choreographed gestures, herbs, crystals, candles, et cetera. It seemed to me that performing spells and rituals was no different from baking: if you follow the step-by-step directions to a T, a successful outcome is likely. I wondered, *What magickal authority gave these occult authors the exact words to string together to make a spell work? How do they know the ritual to make the cute boy in class fall in love with me?* These questions stayed with me, and eventually bothered me enough to the point to where I decided to leave my young witchcraft dreams behind. I decided that magick was a sham; and the cute boy in my class never did fall in love with me, which was the final nail in the coffin!

I don't remember the exact moment or what triggered my eventual understanding, but many years later I came to an empowering realization: the power of magick did not merely reside in assembled words and choreographed movements, but rather in *intention, concentration,* and *energy.* I learned about the law of attraction, the law of sympathy, the law of contagion, hermeticism . . . I connected with other witches and occultists, and things began to fall into place for me. When it came to spellcraft, successful outcomes began to actually happen.

My story of preteen disappointment and eventual epiphany is meant to serve as a reminder that all the rituals and spells you read in this book, or in any book for that matter, are simply suggestions. There are no incantations you must learn word for word and no exact combinations of ingredients or actions that will ensure success in your magick. No matter how etched in stone a spell or ritual seems, they are all open to adaptation. In fact, I encourage you to modify prewritten spells to fit your personal style and needs or make up your own from scratch! They don't have to be fancy or complicated; some of the best spells are short and simple. An elaborate ritual is no good if it has you fumbling over words and steps and worrying about whether you're doing it right. Witchcraft ends with the word *craft* for a reason; it's about creativity and, at the end of the day, it is your will, attitude, and unbroken concentration that work to set the powers that be in motion. Everything else is there to assist you in raising, strengthening, and focusing that energy.

Regarding the well-known rituals used in magick today, especially those of ceremonial magick, such as casting a circle, the lesser and greater banishing rituals of the pentagram, or drawing down the moon, it's important we remember that these rituals were created by humans who were simply using their abilities of creativity and intuition. They felt the energy of the plant or the moon or the season and applied it to what they felt was the proper use. You are capable of the very same. A frequent question I'm asked is, "Do you have a spell for ___?" and my answer is usually, "Yes, but why use mine when you can create your own?" While there are guidelines to spellcrafting, it is my firm opinion that there are no rules.

All that said, I hope that what you find in these pages will help to expand your knowledge of the various esoteric practices and how even the apparently separate ones can work together seamlessly. *Runes for the Green Witch* is organized into twenty-four main chapters—one for every rune of the Elder Futhark. With each one I will present the associated plants and how they have been traditionally used both magickally and medicinally. I have also included various other correspondences such as tarot, planets, and deities to provide you with further ideas should you decide to explore other combinations of magickal synergy; and I encourage you to do so. Learning basic correspondences is a wonderful foundation for those who wish to create their own spells and rituals.

Within this book we will focus on plants and runes, which have much in common. Like each plant, the Norse runes are microcosms that contain within them the blueprints of the macrocosmic. They are both manifestations of cosmic and Earth energies. They are reflections of the dynamic and mysterious forces of nature. While the runes themselves did not grow from the soil as plants did, these ancient symbols are no doubt products of divine interaction with humans, as well as ancient humanity's inability to explain the forces of nature and their fascination with the elements and seasons.

Both runes and plants possess the capacity for healing or harm. To paraphrase famed alchemist Paracelsus, "The difference between medicine and poison is the dose." This important aphorism reminds us to refrain from the temptation of labeling runes, plants, *nature,* as "bad" or "good." Everything has a spectrum. Such generalizations rob these spiritual vessels of their complexities.

Even though there are a mere twenty-four runes compared to the nearly four hundred thousand species of plants on Earth, they both offer infinite uses and wisdom. Both can take us from the mundane to the ecstatic. Both can aid in magick and ritual. Both encompass the primal spirituality of nature. One works to strengthen the other, and the synergy of these two practices equates to a sum far greater than the parts. It was when I combined them that my personal practice began to truly take shape. It was an aha moment, and one that I did not wish to keep to myself. The ultimate purpose of this book is to highlight the strengths of synergistic magick while encouraging a true connection (or reconnection) with the witches' raison d'être: Nature. Through runes and plants, which complement each other beautifully, we will honor the wild spirit that resides in each and every one of us.

THE MAGICK OF PLANTS

We harness the power of plants in a myriad of ways. We consume them, bathe in them, fill our homes and yards with them, burn them as incense, create medicines and magickal blends such as tinctures, potions, ritual oils, and other charms. When it comes to healing, plants can be used for just about anything, from anxiety to dandruff, from indigestion to heartbreak.

If you are brand new to working with herbs or magick in general, you might be wondering how an herb can be used to heal heartbreak. That is an excellent question. Like everything else in nature, plants comprise energies and vibrations that affect the body, mind, and spirit. For ailments of the heart, we can look to the hawthorn tree, which has an affinity for cardiac health. Clinical studies have shown that hawthorn berries benefit the heart in more ways than one. They support muscle toning, improve circulation, reduce strain, and energize cells. These remarkable energies that focus on the physical strengthening of the heart lend themselves equally to the emotional matters of the heart such as love, joy, and grief. There's no doubt that our thoughts affect our health. Think of the physiological symptoms of stress. The heaviness of extreme grief alone can cause a sudden enlargement of the heart muscles, resulting in heart failure. It's a rare condition called *takotsubo cardiomyopathy,* or broken-heart syndrome, and it's just one example of how the different levels that make up the self interact energetically. Engineer and inventor Nikola Tesla once said, "If you want to find the secrets of the universe, think in terms of energy, frequency, and vibration."* And that is precisely how we come to understand the way plants heal, and they do so holistically.

---

*Goodreads (website), "Nikola Tesla > Quotes."

Stress is a low-vibrating response in the mind that radiates low vibrations throughout the physical body. Depression, which affects almost 10 percent of Americans currently, can manifest a slew of physical symptoms such as fatigue, chest pain, muscle aches, headaches, indigestion, and more. Nervousness may cause sweating, and excitement can bring with it a burst of energy. You've probably heard the saying "you are what you eat," and if that's the case then I'm five feet of pizza; but what's equally true (if not more so) is that *you are what you **think***. As the mind, so the body. As above, so below. As the universe, so the soul.

You'll find, as we make our way through the plant profiles, that the magickal and medicinal abilities of a plant tend to overlap. It's not always as clear-cut as they are with hawthorn berries, however. Sometimes the appearance of a plant alone can clue us into its benefits. This is called the *Doctrine of Signatures* and it states that plants resembling various parts of the body can be used to treat ailments of those body parts. It finds similarities between form and function. An example of this is lungwort, which is a plant historically used as a treatment for respiratory ailments such as bronchitis and asthma. Lungwort gets its name from the shape of its leaves, which are said to resemble . . . you guessed it, lungs! Butterfly pea blossoms distinctly resemble a vulva, clitoris and all, and sure enough it may be used to remedy vaginal complaints. It also works well as an aphrodisiac.

As we move through the plant profiles and learn traditional applications in magick and medicine, we must also keep in mind that, just like people, plants are extraordinarily complex. If, in your herbal studies, you find little to no information on the benefits of a certain plant, it isn't because they have none but rather the plant has yet to be examined and documented at length.

It is important to keep in mind that the value of plants go far beyond what magick and maladies they are "good for." Plants are intelligent, spiritual beings. They may not have voices like we do, but they absolutely communicate with us, with their environment, and with each other. To only study plants clinically is to blind ourselves to their wholeness and full potential. We must experience them in nature and listen with spirit, not ears. We'll touch on this more later.

While I prefer a holistic approach to herbalism, I've separated the magickal from the medicinal in the following pages to clearly present the various ways each plant has been worked with throughout antiquity. Once we are given the information, we can then merge the spiritual with the physical and the traditional with the contemporary; we can blur the lines between magick and medicine because truthfully, they're not separate at all.

When learning about a specific plant, I recommend starting by spending one-on-one time with it. One way to do this is by drinking it as a simple infusion (first ensuring it may be safely consumed). A simple infusion is nothing more than a single herb steeped in hot water. Be mindful as you drink it. Focus on the taste, the temperature, and scent. Ask yourself how you feel while ingesting not only the constituents but the spirit of the plant. How do you feel about the herb after drinking it daily for one week? How about two weeks? Learn about its energetic composition, where it typically grows, and its planetary correspondences. Bathe in the herb or burn as incense (again, if these activities are safe with the particular herb). If you feel so inclined, journal about your various experiences with an herb. Did bathing in it feel different energetically than drinking it? These are a few ways to become closely acquainted with plants outside of simply studying them.

The subtle communication between human and plants relies on primal intuition—something many humans today have to work harder to access. In modern times there is a bothersome disconnect between humanity and nature, especially in the West. The more strides humans make in technology, the further we move away from our literal and metaphorical roots. Today, we must try much harder than our ancient ancestors to maintain this connection, as we are faced with endless distractions coming from all directions. When you do find that *something* that strengthens your connection to your roots, I implore you to hang on to it and prioritize it. It's unsettling knowing how easily the spiritual sides of our lives can lose priority to the mundane daily grinds. It's not intentional—we're just overloaded. While the mundane world certainly has its place, it must be balanced with spiritual maintenance. To neglect the spirit is to neglect a large portion of who we are, the part that is eternal and not of this world. Earth is our home, and she's a beautiful, magickal one at that, but she is a temporary home. Those who neglect their spiritual well-being will move through life feeling as though something is missing, like there's a void waiting to be filled. The need for something more flows through our very veins. That need is the reason you find yourself on your current path, the reason you picked up this book.

ELDER FUTHARK RUNES

The following paragraphs comprise a breakdown of the very basics of the Elder Futhark runes and will serve as a primer as we move through the chapters and explore the intricate characteristics of each rune. My hope for those of you who are new to this subject is that you continue to seek knowledge on the history, mythologies, magickal praxis, and theories of the runes.

The word *rune* itself derives from the Gothic *runa* meaning "mystery" or "secret." The word *Futhark* is an acronym made up of the first letter of the first six runes: **Fehu, Uruz, Thurisaz, Ansuz, Raidho,** and **Kenaz.** *Elder* simply distinguishes this set from its successors, the Younger Futhark, which was predominant during the Viking age. This book will focus on the Elder, which is believed to have been created sometime around the first century CE. In modern times, the Elder Futhark remains the most utilized.

The runes of the Elder Futhark possess dual applications—they serve as letters of an "alphabet" and as esoteric spiritual symbols. Because the ancient northerners intimately depended on nature, which, in the winter equated to a potentially hostile environment, the gods and their resulting myths were born out of necessity as a way for folks to deal with and make sense of not-yet-understood natural forces. The runes then provided a channel for open communication between the divine and humans, acting as a language both sides could understand.

The Elder Futhark is made up of twenty-four runes that break down into three groupings of eight called *aettir,* which is the plural form of aett. Each aett is named after a Norse deity and begins with the god's corresponding rune—the first being Freyja's or Freyr's aett, the second, Hagall's aett, and the third, Tyr's aett.

As far as the order of the runes, rest assured it is not arbitrary. The Futhark begins with the themes of creation and birth of all life in the Universe and ends with the personal enlightenment of an individual, similar to the major arcana of the tarot. Each aett represents its own universal theme. Freyja's aett refers to creation, instinct, and basic survival; Hagall's aett represents dynamism, obstacles, and life lessons; and finally, Tyr's aett takes us through social interactions, virtue, and spiritual transformation.

Today, the runes remain a popular method of divination. In most forms of divination, the interpretations deduced from the observed objects rely on how they are drawn. For example, many tarot practitioners apply converse meanings to a card if the image appears upside down. This practice has influenced rune divination, and many modern rune readers will recognize reversed or inverted meanings, aka *murkstave*. Whether you acknowledge reversed meanings is entirely up to you and your intuition.

If you are just learning to work with the runes, I recommend pulling one a day. Read about that rune, carry it with you, meditate on it, and at the end of the day reflect on how it plays a role in your life. Once you become more confident with the meanings, move on to readings of three, then five, and so on. When doing a reading, you may choose to pull them out of a drawstring bag one at a time, toss them onto a cloth, and observe how they land, or if they are all the same shape and color, you can set out all twenty-four face down and intuitively choose three. Another powerful form of rune magick is the art of combining them into sigils called *bindrunes,* which are spells in and of themselves. A bindrune is fashioned of two or more runes, representing the will and intent of the creator. For example, if one is looking to successfully connect and communicate with a fertility goddess, a bindrune of Ansuz and Berkana would be ideal. For safe travel, one might combine Raidho, Kenaz, Ehwaz, and Elhaz. There are countless combinations and uses for them.

Regarding bindrunes, a question I'm often asked by the clients I create them for is "Is it okay that the _____ rune is reversed?" and the answer is yes. Reversed or murkstave runes are not recognized in

bindrunes *unless* that was the intent of the creator. Another common
worry is the inevitable formation of runes that weren't meant to be in
the bindrune. My answer to that is such runes have no power unless
they are given it, otherwise Isa would be present in every bindrune.
Just because Isa can be seen in a bind does not necessarily mean
that the powers of Isa are present in the image. The following figure (below) shows an example of a bindrune that includes both concerns. The intended runes for this particular symbol are Mannaz ᛗ,
Elhaz ᛉ, and Raidho ᚱ and it was created as a general safety (Elhaz)
sigil for a traveling (Raidho) band of musicians (Mannaz). Here we
see some unintended runes such as Gebo ᚷ, Dagaz ᛞ, Hagall ᚼ,
Wunjo ᚹ, Sowilo ᛋ, Kenaz ᚲ, Uruz ᚢ, Teiwaz ᛏ, Ehwaz ᛗ, Eihwaz ᛇ,
Nauthiz ᚾ, Laguz ᛚ, and of course Isa ᛁ. While some of these unin-
tentional runes support the purpose of the overall bindrune such as
Gebo ᚷ, Wunjo ᚹ, and Sowilo ᛋ, others, if chosen deliberately, could
be seen as counterintuitive to its overall goal. That is why the following is so important: a sigil is not empowered by the image itself but
rather by the intention charged into the image as it's created. In this
bindrune we also see a reversed Raidho ᚱ and someone who recog-
nizes reversed (murkstave) runes might mistakenly interpret that as a
sign of misfortune during travel. Again, unless that was the intention
(which in this case, it was not) then its position does not endanger
the objective.

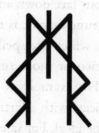

   When it is time to get your own set of runes, I highly recommend
creating your own, especially for your first set. It is believed that the
first runes used for divination were carved onto strips of bark, such as
birch, and many practitioners follow that tradition today. There is no
rule regarding what type of wood they must be made of, however, and

any natural materials will do. Other popular materials are stone, bone, seashells, and clay.

For my personal main set, I created my runes from a fallen branch of a weeping willow, my favorite tree, and quite the magickal one at that. First the branch was placed upon my altar for a full moon cycle and covered with various cleansing and charging items such as herbs, crystals, and charms. Once the moon cycle ended, I began the process of cutting one wooden coin per day.

Day one consisted of sawing a single wooden coin from the willow branch, burning the Fehu stave on one side only, meditating with it, and finally, charging it in a singing bowl with herbs and small crystals where it remained overnight. This I did every day for twenty-four days until all the runes were complete. On day twenty-five I performed an elemental consecration by blessing each rune with a blend of Earth (such as salt, soil, or herbs), incense for Air, a lit candle for Fire, and moon Water, to which I added a few drops of my blood with the help of a sterile lancet. It's common practice for serious rune workers to consecrate and stain their runes with their own blood in order to facilitate a bond between runes and practitioner. For those not comfortable using blood, saliva works great as well. The process described here is my own. Feel free to use and adapt it or create your own entirely; just make sure the process is done with sincerity.

Now that you've been properly introduced to the Elder Futhark runes, we can begin to explore their kinship to the plant kingdom and their various applications in healing, ritual, spellcasting, charms, and connecting to the spirit of nature. I invite you to explore the power of plants and runes with me, as there is much to be discovered.

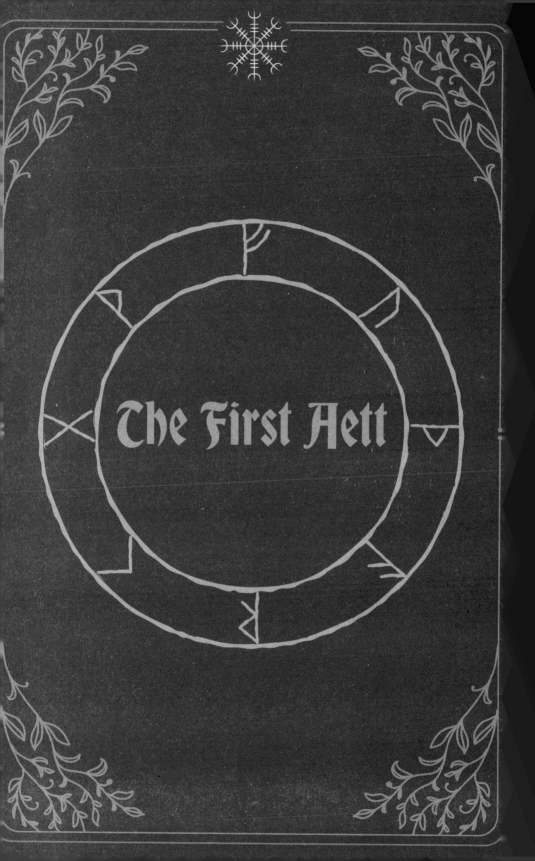

The First Aett

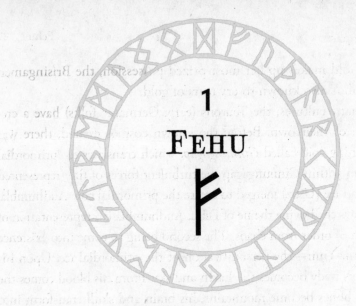

1

FEHU

ᚠ

Phonetic equivalent: F
Finances, Career, Success

Fehu is fortune, luck, and wealth
Hard-earned success and ideal health
It warns to shield oneself from greed
And share one's gains with those in need

We begin our runic journey with Fehu (pronounced fay-hoo), the first rune of the Elder Futhark and Freyja's Aett. In its simplest form it is the rune of money and success—in the early days of the runes, however, it referred mainly to livestock, which was a primary means of currency in many early cultures, including ancient Germanic. The number of livestock owned dictated a person's or family's financial status. Additional meanings of Fehu include career, social status, productivity, fertility, and good health. *Fehu* itself translates to "cattle" and is the root of the English word *fee*.

Within Norse mythology, Fehu is associated with divine siblings Freyja and Freyr, both of whom are deities of fertility. Alongside other fertility gods and goddesses, they reside in Vanaheim, which is one of the nine worlds of which the World Tree is comprised. This tribe of Norse deities is referred to as the Vanir. Freyja's relationship to the rune of wealth is reinforced via her title as a fertility goddess and her affinity for gold. Gold makes up her most prized possession, the Brísingamen necklace. She's also known to cry tears of gold.

Like many cultures, the Teutons (early Germanic folks) have a creation myth of their own. Before the known cosmos existed, there was only a yawning void called *Ginnungagap*, which translates to "primordial abyss." From within Ginnungagap the turbulent forces of fire (represented by Fehu) and ice (Uruz) merged to create the primordial cow Audhumbla, which follows the bovine theme of Fehu. Audhumbla is a representation of the creation of order from chaos. The second being to come into existence was the giant Ymir—the personification of the primordial ice. Upon his death, Ymir's body becomes the Earth and sky. From his blood comes the oceans, his bones become mountains, his brain and skull transform into the clouds and sky, and so on. This is, of course, a very bare-bones version of the story, but from it we can understand better how Fehu can represent different themes from cattle to the creation of the known cosmos.

While Fehu's corresponding element is Fire, it is also a rune of Earth, being associated with the material aspects of life. It does, however, go beyond the simple meanings of money, wealth, and status as any area of life—relationships and health for example—may be prosperous or deprived. Fehu is the reward for honest hard work and perseverance. It serves as a reminder to be grateful for the riches in our lives because they are not promised and can be lost in the blink of an eye.

When considering the meanings of Fehu in a reading, it's important to remember that its revelations are very much reliant on the nature of the inquiry, as well as the surrounding runes in a spread. In readings, Fehu tends toward career aspects, finances, creative endeavors, and beginnings. With Mannaz it may refer to a group enterprise, and alongside Gebo it may indicate the need to share one's wealth or a debt owed. Reversed or murkstave, the wealth rune can indicate greed, envy, financial trouble, ill health, infertility, or lack of creativity. Socially, reversed Fehu can refer to a lowering of status or relationship troubles. Energetically, it seeks to provide abundance while simultaneously warning against greed, materialism, laziness, and overconsumption.

As mentioned previously, Fehu's wealth meaning isn't solely about money, but what holds value in general. Take stock of your life; what is most valuable to you? Common answers typically include the people and animals we love, good health, our homes, family heirlooms, music, art, and so on. If we look a bit deeper, answers may include peace of mind, connection to spirit, intuition, compassion, and honesty, among others.

If it's considered a sacrifice to give something away, then that something has value; and that is how Fehu ties into the importance of offerings. We honor those we revere with items and acts of value. *Acts* of value include rites and ritual, chants, music, dance, and vows of devotion. Offerings are immensely important within magickal practice as it shows we're not just in it for the taking. Not only do I leave offerings for those that assist me but also to possible spirits who may be working against my intentions. It's not far-fetched to think that we may unintentionally offend some beings along the way, especially in the beginning when we're still learning.

As we move through the chapters, we will explore how each rune can support us in the process of rewilding—a journey that helps heal the separation between human and the natural world. Based on its meanings and energies, what are some of the ways Fehu can foster a meaningful connection to nature? One example is the building of outdoor altars. These can be temporary or permanent and are excellent for honoring the Earth and land spirits. It's not even necessary to lug a table outside as boulders and tree stumps are perfect.

An altar may be as simple or as elaborate as one chooses. My only recommendation for what you place on your altar is that items be made entirely of organic materials instead of plastics or any items that would be considered litter if the wind were to displace them. Be careful not to leave anything out that can harm the local wildlife, such as "human foods" that are not available in the wild—especially processed foods. Some options for what you can include on your altar or leave as an offering are runes and other symbols, herbal teas, fresh water, bird seed, flowers and foliage, rocks and crystals, candles, stone statuary—you get the idea.

If creating an outdoor altar is just not possible for you, no worries! I live in the city, so yards aren't really a luxury I have—at least not big yards. One of my favorite ways to honor the Earth is to go outside to either a local park or cemetery and find myself a somewhat secluded spot, preferably under a large tree, where I leave offerings similar to those suggested in the previous paragraph. If you have nothing physical to offer, a silent prayer of gratitude goes a long way. Some folks like to offer pieces of themselves, such as strands of hair or even nail clippings. On the surface these don't seem like items of value, however, every part of our physical being contains a piece of our essence or spirit, which is the most valuable of all.

When it comes to offerings, I've heard more than a few times practitioners voicing concerns over not having items or food that they can part with as offerings, and that's quite understandable. As was briefly pointed out, however, offerings can come in the form of actions. Such actions may include performances like singing and dancing or tasks that support the health and beauty of the Earth, such as picking up litter, consciously reducing waste, walking or biking instead of driving, or planting and maintaining a garden. The power of words and ritual is huge, and through them we can express devotion to the Great Mother without making ourselves go hungry or broke.

Regarding your altar, it's important to remember that it is an extension of the most magickal and sacred of all—you. Your outdoor altar should reflect your practice as well as your relationship to Mother Earth. It represents a place of sanctity where you can honor and convene with the spirits of your environment. The process of building it alone is a ritual in and of itself and is best done mindfully with intention and heart. Hail, Fehu!

CORRESPONDENCES OF FEHU

ELEMENT	Fire, Earth
ZODIAC	Capricorn
PLANET	Jupiter
MOON PHASE	Waxing
TAROT	Ace of Pentacles, 9 of Pentacles
CRYSTAL	Green Aventurine
CHAKRA	Sacral
DEITIES	Fortuna, Freyja, Freyr, Ganesh, Lakshmi, Tsai Shen
PLANTS	Alfalfa, Allspice, Cedar, Cinquefoil, Dandelion, Irish Moss, Peppermint, Rose Hips

The following plants have been chosen for Fehu due to their associations with money and material wealth. When it comes to magick for financial abundance, there is an *abundance* of herbs and plants at your disposal (insert winking face here for nerdy mom joke).

Alfalfa
(*Medicago sativa*)

Alfalfa is an ancient member of the legume family with an affinity for prosperity and abundance. Its energies draw in wealth while simultaneously offering protection against greed and financial crisis. Alfalfa has long been a key source of nutrition for cattle, which as we discussed earlier, was once a primary form of currency; therefore, it is plants such as alfalfa that allowed families to keep healthy livestock and maintain a certain level of status. Keep some inside your wallet, or if you're a business owner, in the cash drawer to attract customers. A simple and effective way to work with alfalfa during abundance rituals is to burn it as incense. To increase the power of such magick, call on the power of Fehu by intoning its name or drawing it on your body; for best results do so on a waxing or full moon. Thursdays are ideal as well, as they're ruled by Jupiter—the planet of expansion. The waxing moon phase is also the best time to harvest alfalfa. Like Fehu, alfalfa not only attracts financial good fortune but also optimal health.

Medicinal Properties

Alfalfa is a moistening nutritive, rich in key vitamins and minerals. Medicinally, it targets arthritis, lack of appetite, debility, mineral deficiencies, indigestion, and it is cleansing to the blood. Use with peppermint for a strong digestive remedy. Alfalfa helps to lower cholesterol, which in turn reduces the risk of heart attack. The high fiber content remedies constipation and reduces gut inflammation. Alfalfa works to improve metabolic health. Actions: anticoagulant, anti-inflammatory, antioxidant, bitter, diuretic, estrogenic, galactagogue, laxative, nutritive, vulnerary. Cooling and moistening. Contraindicated for those who take anticoagulant medications and those with lupus.

Allspice
(*Pimenta officinalis*)

Allspice is a magnet for wealth and success. It is a common food flavoring and can imbue a meal with auspicious energies—an excellent way to promote successful outcomes during business dinners. The dried, powdered berry is great for the coating of candles in money-drawing spells. Whole dried berries may be added to charms and sachets for abundance. Allspice encourages one to feel worthy of success, in turn motivating the practitioner to work harder to achieve their goals. While spells work to make outcomes more likely, it's important we remember as practitioners of magick that we must also do our part in the physical realm to achieve our desires.

Medicinal Properties

Allspice is the dried, unripened berry of the aromatic *Pimenta dioica* tree. The berries contain estrogenic properties that assist in relieving the various symptoms of menopause. Allspice is antifungal and may be used to treat yeast infections. It is a strong digestive used for combating diarrhea, excessive hunger, and flatulence. Colds, fatigue, sore muscles, mild headaches, and menstrual cramps may be remedied with allspice. Actions: analgesic, antibacterial, anticancer, anti-inflammatory, antioxidant, antiseptic, antiviral. Warming. Avoid remedial use during pregnancy.

Cedar
(*Cedrus* spp.)

Cedar is synonymous with strength, pride, and abundance. The tree is said to bring courage during times of struggle and change. Similar to alfalfa, bits of cedar may be added to a wallet or cash drawer to attract a steady flow of funds. Cedar brings with it the powers of protection, not only from harmful forces but from thieves as well. The smoke of cedar incense is cleansing to the aura while charging it with vital energies. The incense also encourages communication with the spirit world. Wands and staffs may be constructed from the wood, but I advise using only fallen branches as causing harm to the tree is said to bring misfortune carried out by the spirits of the land and trees. One of my favorite ways to use cedar is with rosemary for smoke wands. "By Fehu and cedar, wealth I attract. As long as they're with me my money won't lack!"

Medicinal Properties

The essential oil of cedar has a long and diverse history from perfumes to the Ancient Egyptian embalming process. Massaging the diluted essential oil onto the chest helps to relieve congestion. Applied to scalp, cedar encourages hair growth and is especially beneficial in treating alopecia. It also helps reduce dandruff and soothes eczema of the scalp. In aromatherapy, the scent is used to alleviate anxiety and grant strength during crises. Actions: antifungal, antiseptic, antispasmodic, astringent, decongestant, diuretic, expectorant, sedative. Cooling. Avoid internal use. Avoid during pregnancy.

Cinquefoil
(*Potentilla canadensis*)

Cinquefoil, also known as five finger grass, has a diverse history in magick and occult practices. It promotes lucid and prophetic dreaming, especially when used in tandem with dream-enhancing herbs like yarrow, lobelia, or mugwort. With Jupiter's expansive energies at its helm, cinquefoil brings potency to spells for increase and growth. It is believed that the plant is best harvested at midnight under a waxing moon. If you run a brick-and-mortar business, add cinquefoil to floor washes to help increase financial gain. Fun fact: cinquefoil encourages bountiful yields for fishermen, which is great for those of you who prefer an abundance of fish over an abundance of money! (And who doesn't, am I right?)

Medicinal Properties

As a cooling, toning astringent, cinquefoil relieves digestive upsets such as bloating, gas, dysentery, and diarrhea. A mouthwash made from the root soothes mouth sores, sore throats, and toothaches. Traditionally, the root bark has been made into a topical paste to heal wounds, sores, ulcers, bruises, and sunburn. Actions: anti-inflammatory, antispasmodic, astringent, digestive, febrifuge, vulnerary. Cooling and drying.

Dandelion
(*Taraxacum officinale*)

Dandelion grows all over the world and is one of the most recognizable plants. It is a symbol of resilience due to its ability to grow and thrive in conditions unsuitable for most plant life, such as roadsides. These beautiful "weeds" decorate millions of landscapes every spring promising warmer days and more sunshine to come. Whether we knew it or not, many of us have performed magick with dandelions since childhood! This well-known ritual is accomplished by blowing the feathery seeds into the wind, where they can then carry out our secret wishes. Like most solar herbs, dandelion corresponds to health, wealth, and vitality. Money and healing magick are among the variety of ways to use its power. This sunny plant also contains psychic properties and aids in trance and divination. Its roots are especially connected to Samhain, the underworld, and the goddess Hekate.

Medicinal Properties

One of dandelion's most charming folk names is without a doubt "piss the beds," and such a name underlines it strength as a diuretic and detoxifier. While most people wouldn't want to wet the bed or pee their pants, increased urination is beneficial for kidney and urinary infections. Dandelion contains high levels of polyphenols, which are cancer preventatives. These polyphenols, which are at the highest concentration in the flower, also treat cardiovascular diseases, neurodegenerative diseases, diabetes, and osteoporosis. Dandelion also benefits the microflora of the gut. Actions: alterative, anticancer, anti-inflammatory, antioxidant, bitter, cholagogue, detoxifier, digestive, diuretic, hepatoprotective. Cooling. Avoid ingestion of the root if pregnant or breastfeeding. Those with ragweed allergies may become irritated by dandelion.

Irish Moss
(*Chondrus crispus*)

Irish Moss brings good fortune to all matters of money and business. It is a gambler's herb, and one would do well to keep some on their person at the casino. Dried, it may be added to sachets, amulets, and spell jars created to attract money. For owners of brick-and-mortar businesses, grind the dried plant into a powder and periodically sprinkle in each corner of the store as well as the cash drawer.

Medicinal Properties

Irish moss is a nutrient-rich seaweed that doubles as a vegan substitute for gelatin. Its moistening properties relieve dry cough, sore throat, skin irritation, urinary infections, and vaginal dryness. Irish moss contains iodine, which is necessary for healthy thyroid function. Actions: anti-inflammatory, emollient, expectorant, laxative, mucilaginous, nutritive. Cooling and moistening. Those who take blood thinners should avoid Irish moss.

Lady's Mantle
(*Alchemilla vulgaris*)

The Latin name for lady's mantle, *Alchemilla,* comes from the word alchemy, highlighting the plant's ability to increase the power and effectiveness of alchemical processes. This mercurial plant lends itself to the success of magickal workings and is a teacher of the metaphysical arts. As per the name, lady's mantle is feminine in nature and is associated with the goddesses Gaia and Freyja. It is a wonderful ally for those who are trying to conceive. The morning dew found on lady's mantle is thought to be especially potent and may be sprinkled on or under the bed before sex to encourage conception. A bindrune of Fehu and Berkana is a potent symbol for fertility and can be drawn on a leaf of lady's mantle and kept near the bed to increase the chances of becoming pregnant.

Medicinal Properties

As the name implies, lady's mantle has an affinity for feminine health. It is a valued uterine tonic that effectively treats heavy menstrual bleeding, painful menstrual cramping, and vaginal discharge. The hot tea is ideal for soothing cramps and also works well for sore throat and cough. Its astringent properties alleviate diarrhea and speed up the healing time of external wounds. Lady's mantle works to ease allergies, lower cholesterol, and soothe pain caused by endometriosis. Actions: antidiarrheal, antioxidant, antispasmodic, astringent, decongestant, uterine tonic, vulnerary. Drying. Avoid during pregnancy.

Peppermint
(*Mentha piperita*)

Peppermint reminds me of my childhood—specifically that of playing in my nana's garden, which was full of this fresh-scented herb. It was her go-to remedy for upset stomach, and now that I'm a mom (and practitioner of herbal healing), it's one of my go-tos as well. Aside from stomach troubles, peppermint is traditionally applied to money and healing magick, as it works to clear stagnant energies while simultaneously attracting good fortune. Fresh sprigs throughout the home will repel bad luck, mischievous spirits, and evil intent. One whiff of the plant is enough to make one feel refreshed and add a little pep in their step. Add the leaves to a wash for magickal tools or sprinkle around the home to renew energies and raise vibrations. The optimism and vibrancy of this herb also works to attract romance into one's life and can be burned as an aphrodisiacal incense.

Medicinal Properties

Peppermint is aromatic and uplifting and most often used as a tea or essential oil. The carminative properties soothe upset stomach and excess gas. As a tincture, it is best taken between meals to aid in healthy digestion. Peppermint has mild pain-relieving effects that are beneficial for those who suffer with headaches and migraines that come with a side of nausea. It can, however, increase heartburn and symptoms of gastroesophageal reflux disease. Applied as a topical preparation, its antimicrobial qualities help to reduce breakouts while rejuvenating the skin. Actions: analgesic, anesthetic, antibacterial, antiemetic, anti-inflammatory, antioxidant, antiseptic, antispasmodic, antiviral, aromatic, carminative, cholagogue, choleretic, diaphoretic, digestive, diuretic, emmenagogue, expectorant, immunostimulant, nervine, stimulant, stomachic, tonic, vasodilator, vermifuge. Cooling, warming, and drying. Avoid with children under five years of age.

Rose Hips
(*Rosa canina*)

A combination of Taurus and Libra energies make rose hips well suited for both money and love magick. Charge rose hips with intention and add a few in a wallet or money-drawing oil. As a berry of beauty and abundance, it is ideal for ensuring lucrative creative endeavors such as visual arts, performance arts, or writing a book just to name a few. (Yes, I'm fully stocked on rose hips at the moment!) They are also great for adding sweetness and reconciliation to soured situations or relationships.

Medicinal Properties
Rose hips are rich in vitamin C and antioxidants and aid in the absorption of nutrients. They are commonly found in skin care products and are beneficial (and yummy) additions to cold, flu, and fever remedies. Due to their astringent properties, rose hips are great for "wet" colds, especially, as they help to dry up excess phlegm. Half a teaspoon of rose hip syrup is a pleasantly sweet way to ease teething pain in babies. They are also a wonderful additive in remedies for osteoarthritis. Actions: antibacterial, anti-inflammatory, antioxidant, astringent, nutritive. Neutral.

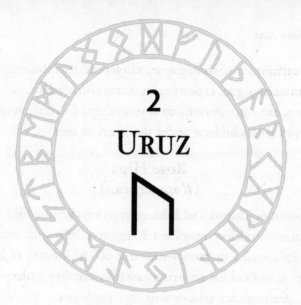

2
URUZ

ᚢ

Phonetic equivalent: U
Strength, Energy, Health

The aurochs stands a mighty beast
Unmatched in primal strength
It reigns supreme within the wild
A force lacking constraint

Next in line is the mighty Uruz (pronounced ew-rooz), the rune of the long-horned aurochs—an extinct species of large wild cattle comparable in size to the modern bison. The Roman author Tacitus informs that the killing of an aurochs served as a rite of passage into manhood for young Germanic men.

With Fehu we discussed domesticated cattle, while with Uruz we meet their untamable relatives. Like the aurochs Uruz represents strength, endurance, and ferocity. When I visualize the meaning of this rune I tend toward the "bull in a china shop" analogy. It also brings to mind the animalistic nature of humanity that remains mostly caged and hidden from society. Uruz contains a wild, palpable energy. While it typically calls to mind physical strength, it may just as well indicate mental or spiritual strength. In the Norse myth of creation, Uruz represents the primordial ice that meets with Fehu's fire to inaugurate the chaotic event that launched existence; what modern science refers to as the big bang. The prefix *Ur-* means "proto" or "original."

Uruz is a rune of vitality and often applies to healing. Both Uruz and Sowilo, the sun rune, are amazing healing runes. When a fellow rune worker in my community came down with COVID, she performed a healing ritual, during which she drew Uruz on both sides of her chest over her lungs. When my elderly dachshund hurt his leg, I wrapped the injured leg in gauze inscribed many times with the rune while repeating a healing incantation (along with a trip to the vet). As an herbalist, Uruz is a rune I work with often. Most herbal remedies that I create are blessed and charged with the healing powers and vitality of Uruz and Sowilo.

If you're feeling drained and in need of energy, Uruz is like the coffee of runes, although it doesn't come with the dreaded jitters and crash of caffeine! When I feel like I'm too tired to start my day, I trace Uruz over my head, heart, and stomach with an invigorating oil and envision a burst of energy within.

As a rune of primitive energy, Uruz corresponds to the root chakra, which is the energy center of instinct, survival, and sex. This rune is also helpful in the clearing of a blocked throat chakra, as it can help one assert themselves and reclaim their voice; especially when paired with Ansuz. Just like in the healing rituals mentioned previously, Uruz may be drawn over the throat during chakra meditation or simply when one is looking for the courage to speak their mind. Some of us have grown up in households, communities, or countries that do not allow their members to speak out truthfully, under the threat of severe consequences. Uruz is an ally for those who refuse to stay silent and oppressed. Do not take this to mean that I consider silence to be a weakness, because in many situations, it's a true means of survival. I would never encourage anyone to place themselves in a dangerous situation. Those who have moved beyond the constraints of strict families or communities may need a bit of help once they are ready to speak up, and Uruz is a wonderful rune to have at one's side.

Like a bull in a china shop, Uruz does come with an inherent element of chaos, but that's not necessarily a bad thing. The wild rune is related to the chaotic creation of the cosmos. While formidable and fast-paced, its energies contain a sense of neutrality. Most stories of creation are essentially stories of something being made from nothing— the ultimate manifestation. Therefore, Fehu and Uruz together may be employed as a bindrune when one is trying to manifest within their own practice or life. There is enormous momentum packed within this rune, and it's a helpful token for those who tend to procrastinate or simply need a little push.

In matters of romance, Uruz represents lust and sexuality. It's the initial spark between two people. It's fiery and passionate, but on the other side of that coin it's potentially explosive and disorderly. Other related meanings are determination, hard work, and raw power. Murkstave, Uruz may indicate physical or emotional weakness, lack of willpower, anxiety, destruction, or illness.

Uruz is an ally for those reconnecting to Mother Earth due to its primitive nature. This healing rune aids in the process of revealing the authentic inner self by peeling back the many layers of beliefs, agreements, and ideologies we adopt over time. It takes us back to factory settings. *Rewilding* has become a popular term for this. The environmental definition describes rewilding as the restoration of land to its natural state. So how do we, as humans, rewild and return to our natural states? My initial thought was, get naked in the forest, *obviously;* and hey, that's one way to get wild for sure, but sadly it isn't an option for many of us. (It's quite tragic, really.) Meditating outdoors, preferably in a natural area, is a great place to start (and if you're going to do it naked, bring a blanket to sit on. Twigs—ouch!).

Begin by finding a private spot, or if sitting isn't possible, walking meditation works, too. Focus on the sounds you hear, the way the Earth feels below you, the smell of the fresh air, and the sight of your surroundings. Remember that you are not an outsider to your surroundings; you are *part* of it all. Through meditation and breathwork, find your rhythm with the Earth below and around you. If I'm sitting, I like to place my palms on the earth and call up her energy into me. Do your best to be present, and if you find your mind drifting to your to-do list or the things you *should've* said during your last argument, gently bring your attention back to your senses and how they are experiencing your current environment. Listen to the birds and feel the wind on your skin. Visualize tree roots growing out from you and digging deep down into the Earth, anchoring you. Visualize branches growing out from your shoulders and head, reaching up into the sky, past the clouds, all the way to the stars. Green chthonic energy from the Earth courses up through the roots while gold and silver celestial energy courses down through the branches, together merging at your heart center and filling you with glowing warmth. Experience this for as long as you'd like. When you feel that you are finished, offer gratitude to the Earth, the sky, and to yourself. This is a great practice not only for connecting to nature but also for gathering energy before performing magick.

Rewilding is a major theme of this book, and it's a personal journey that looks different for everyone. In the previous chapter of Fehu, we discussed the power of offerings and outdoor altars. If any rune were to represent rewilding it would, without a doubt, be Uruz. It's easy for us humans to forget that we were once wild animals, and really, we still are—the part of us we tend to keep cloaked under layers of social constructs.

Rewilding the spirit takes time and patience and the willingness to leave one's comfort zone. For many of us, leaving home without a phone is cause for anxiety, when it wasn't all that long ago that our giant phones were connected to the wall by an electrical cord. Once I was watching a movie set in the eighties with my twelve-year-old son, and he was dumbfounded by the contraption with the curly cord that people talked into! It's fun explaining to modern young folks that life in the eighties and nineties, though not so long ago, was much different. *You had to wait an entire week to watch the next episode of a TV show?!* That's right, streaming has not been available since the dawn of time.

Now that we have the luxuries of smart phones, leaving such technologies behind is not so easy. We grow attached to such conveniences. Even when we're not actively using our smart phones, they are still emitting radiation that we inevitably absorb. If part of your rewilding experience includes breaks from technology, don't just turn off your smart phone, put it away in a drawer. It's helpful to begin such practices in small increments of time, like during walks, and eventually working your way up to a weekend camping trip sans technological devices.

The following is an example of an incantation I use to evoke Uruz for aid with rewilding. Typically, I recite this before an outdoor meditation like the one previously described, but it can be used and adapted to fit your own needs:

> *I call on the mighty Uruz*
> *Powers of creation and chaos*
> *Please guide me as I seek out*
> *My primal roots and truth*
> *Please guide me as I seek a*
> *Deeper connection to the Earth*
> *For I was born of Earth and*
> *Upon my death I will return*

Hail, Uruz!

CORRESPONDENCES OF URUZ

ELEMENT	Ice
ZODIAC	Aries
PLANET	Mars
MOON PHASE	Waxing
TAROT	The Fool, Knight of Wands
CRYSTAL	Blue Aventurine
CHAKRA	Root
DEITIES	Aja, Chiron, Hercules, Kali, Kratos
PLANTS	Agrimony, Bay Laurel, Echinacea, Eucalyptus, Ghost Pipe, Juniper, Pau D'Arco, Rue

The energies of Uruz are complex, as are the plants that correspond to the rune of strength. The plants of Uruz capture the spirits of healing, primitive wildness, and fortitude of the mind, body, and soul.

Agrimony
(*Agrimonia eupatoria*)

Agrimony is an aggressive defender of spirit, touted for its abilities to protect from and reverse psychic attacks. This member of the rose family has an affinity for the energy body and may be used to cleanse, heal, and reinforce the auric field. To gain deep, rejuvenating rest while repelling nightmares, bathe in agrimony prior to sleep and/or place some dried leaves under a pillow. Combine with hops or jasmine to enhance its restful effects. This calming quality helps to aid one in achieving a deep state of trance. When agrimony teams up with Uruz the result is a formidable force against malevolence, bad luck, and illness. When ill or injured, the smoke of agrimony incense is helpful in clearing stagnant energies that slow the recovery process. Once the incense has burned out, use the ashes to trace Uruz over the afflicted body part to encourage speedy healing.

Medicinal Properties

As a topical remedy, agrimony benefits various complaints. It may be applied as a compress for migraines and sprains, added to a face-washing regimen to reduce oiliness and acne, or used as an eyewash for conjunctivitis. Agrimony treats wounds and halts excessive bleeding. Make a simple infusion to use as mouthwash for sore throats or canker sores. Taken internally, it targets diarrhea, urinary tract infections, balances the nervous system, and promotes detoxification of the liver and gallbladder. Actions: antibacterial, antiedemic, anti-inflammatory, antioxidant, astringent, expectorant, hepatic, styptic, vulnerary. Drying. Those who take blood thinners or blood pressure medications should not use agrimony. Avoid during pregnancy and nursing.

Bay Laurel
(*Laurus nobilis*)

Today bay leaves are used primarily for culinary reasons but have not fallen out of popular use within metaphysical communities. Historically, crowns woven from bay leaves and branches were gifted as symbols of honor and accomplishment. In fact, the term *bachelor's degree* evolved from *baccalaureate* or *bacca lauri,* which refers to the crown of bay leaves that was often bestowed upon the victorious. Bay is a healer and protector, capable of soothing mental unrest such as anxiety. To aid in the increase of physical or emotional strength, draw Uruz on the skin with a simple blend of olive oil and ground bay leaves while focusing on your goal. The following is a common and simple banishing ritual: On a dry bay leaf write the name of a person, thing, or habit you wish to be rid of. Burn the leaf in a cauldron or other fire-safe receptable and envision the smoke carrying away that which you wish to be free of. And so it is.

Medicinal Properties

Bay is rich in vitamin C and minerals. It works to settle an upset stomach and stimulate appetite, bring on menstruation, and lower bad cholesterol. Bay vapor combats chest congestion and coughs. Apply a topical oil or poultice to treat bruising, sprains, arthritis, muscle pain, and joint pain. Actions: antibacterial, antifungal, anti-inflammatory, carminative, diaphoretic, digestive, emetic, emmenagogue, nutritive, stimulant, vermifuge. Warming. When working with the essential oil for the first time, be sure to dilute and test a drop on the skin, as it may cause skin irritations for some.

Echinacea
(*Echinacea purpurea*)

There's far more information available on the health benefits of echinacea compared to its esoteric uses, and such instances leave us with the opportunity to learn from the spirit of the plant directly. Some of the known magickal uses of echinacea include burning it to improve concentration prior to ritual or meditation and the ability to amplify spell work. Echinacea makes for a wonderful offering as a tea, an incense, an amulet, or by itself in a small offering bowl. Because it is so strongly associated with optimal health, it is the perfect addition to any sort of healing magick. In my experience, I've personally found that its energies are quite motivational and fearless—much like the mighty Uruz itself!

Medicinal Properties

During cold and flu season echinacea is a highly sought-after herbal remedy. Not only does it help to prevent the onset of illness, but it also works to relieve symptoms and speed up the recovery process in those who are already sick. Echinacea is one of the first herbs I reach for when I feel under the weather, typically as tea or tincture. The first time I took the tincture I was alarmed by a tingling and numbing sensation on my tongue. I later learned that the feeling is the result of alkamides present in the root, and the feeling is an indication of the plant's potent healing qualities. Echinacea stimulates digestion, increases white blood cells, eases toothaches and sore throats (due to the numbing alkamides), treats viral and fungal infections, and supports liver health. Traditionally, it has been given in response to snakebites, both internally and externally. Actions: alterative, anti-inflammatory, antiseptic, antivenomous, antiviral, detoxifier, immunostimulant, lymphatic, vulnerary. Cooling and drying. Usage should be limited to one to two weeks at a time.

Eucalyptus
(*Eucalyptus* spp.)

Eucalyptus is energizing, revitalizing, and all-around uplifting. It supports optimal health by way of cleansing, purifying, strengthening, and protecting. Because of such energies, it's common to see dried eucalyptus bunches adorning the inside of homes. To provide epic levels of energetic cleansing, anoint a person, place, or object with eucalyptus oil while intoning "Uruz" repeatedly. The intonation adds an extra layer of cleansing via sound vibration. For cleansing space, burn the dried leaves or add a few drops of eucalyptus essential oil to a spray bottle and proceed to bless each corner of the room(s) with the smoke or spritz. When making cleansing mists, moon-, snow-, and rainwater are ideal bases. Include any other cleansing herbs or oils you may have on hand—some suitable options include hyssop, angelica, and frankincense.

Medicinal Properties

The scent of eucalyptus alone is healing and uplifting. Its powerful antiseptic and expectorant qualities make for an excellent herbal remedy for colds, and it is often added to over-the-counter products like lozenges and cough medicine. By dilating the bronchioles, eucalyptus helps to relieve respiratory stress, and it is typically combined with camphor and peppermint in external decongesting ointments. The tea may be used as a gargle for sore throats but refrain from ingesting it as eucalyptus is toxic. Actions: analgesic, antioxidant, antiseptic, bronchodilator, expectorant, stimulant. Warming and drying. Not recommended for daily use.

Ghost Pipe
(*Monotropa uniflora*)

The haunting ghost pipe perennial is quite unique in that it lacks chlorophyll and obtains its energy parasitically from fungi and trees rather than from the sun; this is the reason for its ghostly complexion. This elusive plant is a skillful healer of pain, both emotionally and physically. It helps to ease the overactive mind, clearing away anxiety and worry, and is an ally for folks whose chaotic minds get in the way of effective meditation, ritual, or general day-to-day life. Ghost pipe, also known as corpse plant or Indian pipe, is very rare, and it's recommended that if found to leave it be. Due to its very specific environmental requirements, it is impossible to transplant. If found, simply meditating or working alongside the plant is enough to engage in and use its magickal healing energies.

Medicinal Properties
Alone or combined with other pain-relieving (analgesic or anodyne) herbs, ghost pipe targets moderate to severe pain such as migraines. Its potent nervine and sedative properties aid in relieving panic and anxiety. In the past, it has been used as a remedy for epileptic seizures and fevers. Ghost pipe resembles a brain stem and, true to the doctrine of signatures, helps to regulate the nervous system. Actions: analgesic, antispasmodic, diaphoretic, hypnotic, nervine, sedative. Cooling. Avoid operating vehicles as ghost pipe may cause drowsiness.

Juniper
(*Juniperus communis*)

Juniper is strongly purifying, associated with good health and well-being. It provides comfort and healing after long bouts of illness or substance abuse. Juniper incense repels malevolent spirits who thrive on the energies of others. It effortlessly raises vibrations and works to keep illness at bay. Traditionally the branches were hung in barns to protect the animals from predators, illness, and baneful magick. In Scotland, it's common practice to burn the branches as a New Year's ritual to promote a fresh start and good fortune in the coming year. Any part of the tree can be added to personal charms to attract positive energies and offer protection. One way to create such a charm is by constructing a bracelet or keychain from the berries using a sewing needle and thread. Welsh lore states that one who cuts down the juniper tree will die within a year's time.

Medicinal Properties

Juniper berries are rich in vitamin C and antioxidants. They are ideal for kidney and urinary health due to their strong antiseptic properties. They help to bring on menstruation and have antidiabetic properties. Topical remedies made from the berries and branches ease chronic arthritis. It was once used as a birth control method, but over time it was replaced by safer, more effective methods. It also works as an insect repellant. Actions: antidiabetic, antifungal, anti-inflammatory, antiseptic, aromatic, carminative, diuretic, emmenagogue, kidney tonic, stomachic. Warming and drying. Avoid during pregnancy and nursing. Use with caution in persons with inflammatory kidney disease. Not for long-term use.

Pau D'Arco
(*Tabebuia avellanedae*)

Pau d'arco is native to Central and South America. It is strongly supportive of feminine confidence and sovereignty. One's menstrual cycle should be a source of personal power and connection to the lunar cycles rather than one of debility and misery as it can be for many. Uruz paired with pau d'arco (which counteracts the pain, weakness, and low mood that often accompany menstruation) helps one reclaim that power—especially when working such magick within sight of the moon! Pau d'arco carries energies of inspiration, vibrancy, and prosperity. It is said that the Vikings traded for this herb during their travels to South America as they were enchanted by its uniquely vibrant auburn color.

Medicinal Properties

As an antibiotic and antifungal, pau d'arco is a potent remedy for the treatment of yeast and staph infections. Folks suffering from chronic fatigue may benefit from its plant medicine as well. Pau d'arco helps to prevent and treat stomach ulcers. In ancient South America, it was a go-to medicine for snake bites. Actions: alterative, antibacterial, anticancer, antifungal, anti-inflammatory, antiparasitic, astringent, immunostimulant. Cooling and drying. Avoid alongside blood clotting disorders. High doses may trigger nausea and vomiting. Avoid during pregnancy.

Rue
(*Ruta graveolens*)

Rue has an extensive, compelling history of lore and use throughout various folk traditions. One must only refer to its other common names, *mother of herbs* or *herb of grace,* to understand the long-held reverence of this plant. In Sicilian tradition, rue was used in a popular talisman called the *cimaruta,* a charm that was worn around the neck to protect the wearer from the evil eye and witchcraft (ironic since rue is a popular staple in the witch's apothecary). In ancient Greece, it was regarded as an antidote for illness brought on by hex or curse. Rue is sacred to the goddess of witches, Hekate, as well as Diana and Mars. Fortifying and purifying, this Balkan native is valued for health and healing magick, as well as exorcism and banishing. It helps to strengthen one's psychic abilities. In Europe, people believed it prevented plague. An arrow rubbed with the herb was said to never miss its target. Together, Uruz and rue are an indomitable pair deserving of a celebrity name amalgam—Ruruz! Both are associated with strength, health, and protection, and when used together, the synergy is undeniably raw and commanding!

Medicinal Properties

Historically, rue was given for a multitude of ailments including respiratory complaints, pleurisy, earaches, muscle spasms, hepatitis, epilepsy, and multiple sclerosis. The leaves may be applied topically as a poultice to alleviate headache and sciatic nerve pain, although this should be done with caution as rue may cause adverse skin reactions. As an emmenagogue it works to bring on menstruation; therefore it should never be used during pregnancy or while nursing. It eliminates parasitic worms. Gargle the tea to ease a sore throat. Actions: anti-inflammatory, antispasmodic, emmenagogue, stimulant, vermifuge. Warming. Because rue can cause skin irritation, wear gloves while handling it. Rue may exacerbate gastrointestinal issues. Avoid while pregnant or nursing. It is poisonous in large doses.

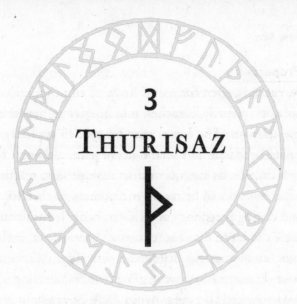

3
THURISAZ

Phonetic equivalent: Th
Defense, Conflict, Unconscious Forces

The fearsome fighter Thurisaz calmly waits to be
  approached
A giant stirring in the shadows, perched to strike
  when danger's close
Thurisaz won't seek you out for battle if there is no
  need
But if you challenge it, its thorns cut deep, and you
  will surely bleed

Thurisaz (pronounced thor-iss-ahz) is third in the Elder Futhark and represents the explosive result of the merging of Fehu's fire and the ice of Uruz. When these two elements make contact within the yawning void of Ginnungagap, chaos ensues, triggering the commencement of the known cosmos. *Thurisaz* translates to "giant" in Proto-Germanic. In Norse mythology, giants are personifications of the forces of nature. Thurisaz is associated with the hammer-wielding god Thor, as the name *Thurisaz* itself is an archaic name for Thor.

Thurs- is the root of the word *Thursday,* the day of the week dedicated to Thor. Energetically, Thursdays are best for invoking the powers of the god of thunder as well as the planet and Roman god, Jupiter. It is an auspicious day for workings of protection, strength, storm energy, expansion, luck, and consecration.

Thurisaz is a rune of defense and is known as the "thorn" rune, which is made evident by its shape. Like a thorn, Thurisaz is mostly passive and does not seek out conflict, but one should think twice before mishandling either. It is a rune of conflict, blood, conception, empowerment, chthonic energy, and hidden consciousness. From the Norwegian and Icelandic rune poems, we can gather that it corresponds to menstruation, as it's described as the illness or torment of women. Some view this rune as a powerful defender, while others see it as a curse. Like any weapon, we can choose to wield it for attack or holster its power until we require it for defensive purposes. It's all about intention. It's important to refrain from labeling runes "bad" or "good," because like people or plants, they are extremely complex. In its most simplistic form, I see Thurisaz as a means of defense. I keep a large Thurisaz that I've constructed from branches hanging on my front porch to ward off those with harmful intentions and energies. While I tend to employ the thorn rune as a magickal form of protection, there's no doubt that this is among the ideal runes for cursing and hexing. As the rune of Thor, it's often likened to his hammer *Mjolnir,* which brandishes the abilities to destroy or heal. Instead of thinking of it as a force of good or evil, perhaps it's best to simply recognize the immense power it contains—a power that must be used wisely and with the utmost care.

Thurisaz is the "take no shit" rune and manifests itself through our instinctual desire to defend ourselves and the people, animals, places, and things we care about. In nature it is a thorny bush, the needles of a cactus, stinging nettles, and poisonous plants. In the animal kingdom it is the venom of a spider, the repellant odor of a skunk, or the sting of a wasp. In modern times we have locks on our doors, security systems, surveillance cameras, and some may have guns. This is all Thurisaz manifest. My dog Lunar is Thurisaz with paws. He is such a sweetheart, but I'd hate to be the intruder who breaks into my house.

In a reading, Thurisaz tends to come as an indication of conflict or as a warning. The nature of the conflict or warning depends on the rest of the spread as well as the order of the runes drawn. Psychologically,

Thurisaz represents a person's deep unconscious—their shadow self—and in this way the rune can be a wonderful ally for those on the journey of spiritual alchemy. Paired with Mannaz it may indicate a rift between parties or the need to be on the defense from others. With Fehu it may warn against mishandling finances or the lowering of one's status. Reversed Thurisaz symbolizes aggression, anger, and mental instability.

One way we can use Thurisaz in the rewilding process is through the exploration of the poison path, or veneficium. The poison path is the branch of herbology that focuses on the study and magick of entheogens and poisonous plants as well as certain species of fungi. Because of their abilities to alter consciousness, disorient, harm, or even kill, these plants are also commonly referred to as "baneful" plants.

In matters of spirit, such plants have an affinity for the shadow aspects of one's personality. The legends and lore associated with baneful plants (or simply, *banes*) often speak of abilities that hex or harm, but it's important to remember they are much more than weaponized plants. Banes are also great healers, especially for traumas and toxicities of the spirit. Due to their connection with death, they cultivate necessary endings that catalyze rebirths and new beginnings. Many of the banes, particularly entheogens, are the shamans of the green world, and have long been escorting witches and mystics past the veil that separates our physical realm from all the others. A few examples of these include psilocybin mushrooms, ayahuasca, and peyote.

Like Thurisaz, banes possess their own defense mechanisms that can cause unwanted side effects to those who consume or even handle them. These mechanisms protect them from being fed on by animals and microorganisms. Taking the time to learn about baneful plants teaches us the neutrality of nature and how concepts of good and evil are essentially man-made constructs.

Many plants of the poison path, such as deadly nightshade, datura, and henbane, have offered medicinal applications throughout history, these uses having fallen away with the increased availability of pharmaceuticals. It's important to keep in mind also that many seemingly benign plants can be dangerous if the dose is high enough, and many of the plants classified as *poisonous* are safe and medicinal if the dose is low enough. Thorough research of each plant and proper dosing knowledge are absolutely essential to successfully working hands on in the poison path or with plant medicine in general.

You may be thinking to yourself *I'm not messing with any poisonous plants,* and trust me, I get it. As the proud owner of a brain that likes to explore all the ways a scenario can go wrong, I tend to exclude most of these from my practice (except psilocybin). When I first started learning about baneful plants, I accidentally grazed a datura flower with my bare hand and just about spiraled into a paranoid panic attack, thinking I had just poisoned myself and was on the brink of death. Turned out I was completely fine, my only symptom being embarrassment from my overreaction. That datura flower now sits atop my Dark Moon altar safely ensconced in a sealed glass jar where I can communicate with it and work with it without having to actually handle it. While I may not include most banes in my green witchery, I'm still an enthusiast. *It is extremely important that banes remain unhandled* until the proper training and knowledge on how to do so safely has been acquired.

Plants of the poison variety are not the only kind that fall under the category of the defense rune. There are many common herbs and spices that are safe to consume and are simultaneously impressive in their abilities to defend; many we will discuss in the following plant profiles.

One thing all the Thurisaz plants have in common is that they're *no nonsense!* These are the plants that aid in cursing and hexing, *breaking* curses and hexes, powerful protection, and banishings—and they bring a big old heaping mound of *don't fuck with me*. When we explore the poison path and Thurisaz together, we are able to see that plants, especially baneful ones, and humans aren't so different after all—at the end of the day we're all just trying to live our lives and not get eaten! Hail, Thurisaz!

CORRESPONDENCES OF THURISAZ

ELEMENT	Fire
ZODIAC	Scorpio
PLANET	Saturn
MOON PHASE	Waning
TAROT	9 of Wands
CRYSTAL	Black Tourmaline
CHAKRA	Solar Plexus
DEITIES	Heimdall, Hekate, Kali, Set, Shiva, Thor
PLANTS	Black Pepper, Cayenne Pepper, Devil's Claw, Dill, Fennel, Garlic

The corresponding herbs of Thurisaz embody the confidence, ferocity, and authority necessary for defense, conflict resolution, and baneful magick. They help to instill a sense of assertiveness within their allies. Many of the following herbs and spices are commonly available in one's kitchen or local grocery. As we'll see below, plants don't have to contain poison to defend against potential threats.

Black Pepper
(*Piper nigrum*)

Black pepper is the ultimate Thurisaz herb. Its Saturnal energies are confident, strong, and able to shield from enemies and harmful energies. It is staunchly defensive against hexes and curses. Black pepper is ideal in magickal workings for protection, exorcism, creating boundaries, and for the ceasing of gossip and jealousy. To ensure that an unwelcome guest never again returns, sprinkle some in their shoes or coat pocket (and don't forget to be sneaky about it!) before they go on their merry way. A small bowl of whole peppercorns makes a great offering for deities that aggressively defend and protect.

Medicinal Properties

Black pepper is one of the most commonly used spices on Earth. Besides adding flavor, it gets the digestive system moving like a well-oiled machine and alleviates minor complaints such as nausea, bloating, constipation, and excess gas. Its active compound, piperine, reduces inflammation, kills bacteria, and provides potent antioxidants to help reverse cellular damage. Historically, it served as a remedy for vertigo. The essential oil helps to alleviate rheumatic pain and muscle tension. It is prominent within ayurveda and traditional Chinese medicine due to its digestive benefits. Actions: antibacterial, antioxidant, antiseptic, carminative, circulatory stimulant, digestive. Warming and drying. Large doses may trigger gastrointestinal upset.

Cayenne Pepper
(*Capsicum frutescens*)

Cayenne pepper is the main ingredient of pepper spray for a reason, and that is its natural ability to sting and repel! It's the perfect additive for banishings, spell jars, hexing, and tacos. Whole peppers hung in the home work to dissipate tension building between loved ones and work to soothe anger. Like black pepper, cayenne helps to ensure an unwanted guest never returns—simply toss a handful out the door behind them as they depart. If someone is pestering you and won't leave you alone, blow a handful of cayenne and black pepper on a photo of them (this is best done outdoors). Burn the photo and discard the ashes far away from your home.

Medicinal Properties

Cayenne contains capsaicin, the compound responsible for its spicy flavor. Capsaicin also serves as a local stimulant and helps alleviate nerve pain and arthritis. Like any heating herb, cayenne works well to improve circulation. Its antimicrobial properties have proved to be a potent remedy against gastroenteritis, also known as the stomach flu. On an emotional level, it is suitable in magickal workings regarding healing shock and trauma. Actions: analgesic, antiseptic, antispasmodic, carminative, circulatory stimulant, diaphoretic, rubefacient, tonic. Warming and drying. Large doses may cause irritation to the stomach and bowels.

Devil's Claw Root
(*Harpagophytum procumbens*)

The energies of devil's claw root are aligned with the planet Mars and therefore fiercely protective in nature. Traditionally, bits of the root are placed in entryways to disorient approaching enemies or pesky solicitors. Burning the root upon moving into a new home clears away residual energies left by the previous occupants. It is an ideal fumigator for before and after magick, particularly practices like necromancy or any kind of spirit interaction where a little extra armor is necessary. Sadly, devil's claw is currently endangered and should be substituted if possible.

Medicinal Properties

Devil's claw, which is an African native, is a prized anti-inflammatory and has been used for thousands of years as a pain reliever for back pain, joint pain, and arthritis. It supports the health of ligaments, tendons, and bones. As a bitter it stimulates digestion and promotes the absorption of nutrients. Devil's claw helps to balance blood sugar. It is known to cleanse the blood and relieve fevers. Actions: antiarthritic, anti-inflammatory, analgesic, bitter, digestive. Cooling and drying. Those who take blood thinners, suffer from heart rhythm disorders, IBS, GERD, or from stomach ulcers should avoid taking devil's claw root. Those who are pregnant or nursing should consult with a healthcare professional.

Dill
(*Anethum graveolens*)

Dill is an herb of protection magick applied often to rituals for banishing or blessing. Like rue, dill is traditionally applied to defend against curses and baneful magick. Sprinkle the seeds at entryways and windows of your home or business to keep away those with ill intentions. Added to a pillowcase, it targets nightmares and encourages peaceful dreams. Add a pinch under the beds of children for safe keeping or include in a protection spell jar or sachet and hide it in their room. Dill brings clarity and mental strengthening. Before calling on dill's protective powers, charge the herb via intonations of Thurisaz. Fehu also works well with dill as they both share an affinity for abundance and fortune.

Medicinal Properties

The name *dill* derives from the Norse word *dylla,* which means "to soothe." Few know of this herb's talents outside of flavoring foods, but aside from making a mean pickle, it's also a handy remedy for a variety of digestive upsets as well as encouraging breast milk production. Dill contains calcium and may help prevent loss of bone density. In ancient Egypt, it was valued for its ability to relieve pain, especially in cases of menstrual discomfort. Actions: analgesic, antidiarrheal, anti-inflammatory, antispasmodic, antirheumatic, aromatic, carminative, digestive, mild diuretic, emmenagogue, galactagogue, immunostimulant, stomachic. Warming.

Fennel
(*Foeniculum vulgare*)

Fennel is a fierce guardian of spirit. It protects against baneful magick of any kind. Like a mirror, it deflects psychic attacks and returns the harmful energies to sender. It's basically the "I'm rubber, you're glue" of protective plants. In times of danger, fennel helps one find the courage and confidence needed to defend themselves and loved ones. It may be employed as incense or as a liquid cleanser to clear and renew a space that's clogged with stagnant heavy energy. It works to open the third eye chakra and help the seer make sense of what is "seen." Drink hot fennel tea to encourage healthy communication or to help with the clearing of a blocked throat chakra.

Medicinal Properties

Today, fennel is primarily used in cooking or as a garnish and has a similar flavor to licorice. Its medicinal properties should not be ignored, however. Just as fennel works well to clear stagnant energy from spaces, it's also great for "clearing out" the body; it's a carminative (relieves flatulence) and a diuretic and helps to break up and pass kidney stones. Combine with catnip to treat colic and other digestive troubles in infants. Fennel not only encourages the flow of break milk but also sweetens it. Actions: antispasmodic, aromatic, carminative, digestive, diuretic, expectorant, galactagogue, mild laxative. Warming and drying. Use cautiously during pregnancy.

Garlic
(*Allium sativum*)

As an Italian with a deep love for nineties vampire television and movies, I'm no stranger to the benefits of garlic. It's as healthy and flavorful as it is a potent ally for protection. Since antiquity it has been valued for its ability to ward off psychic attack and break curses. In general, it's a threatening repellant for harmful energies of any kind, not just vampires! In the homes of some of my family members, it's common to see ropes of garlic hanging in kitchens or entryways to protect the home and family from ill health, wicked entities, and sub-par pasta sauce. The synergy of garlic and Thurisaz is immensely defensive and an intimidating, no-nonsense psychic warning for any ill-intentioned entities that try to come your way.

Medicinal Properties
Garlic is an exceptional healer, capable of treating a variety of ailments as well as maintaining balanced health. Among its talents are the abilities to treat asthma, cold, flu, respiratory infections, ear infection, high cholesterol, and high blood pressure. When I feel like I may be coming down with something, garlic is one of the first items I reach for. Combined with mullein it makes a strong yet gentle respiratory tonic that is suitable for children. Actions: antibacterial, anticoagulant, antidiabetic, antifungal, antiparasitic, circulatory stimulant, decongestant, diaphoretic, expectorant, vermifuge. Warming and drying. Individuals with weakened constitutions should avoid garlic. To prevent gastric irritation, take with or after meals. It may exacerbate heartburn.

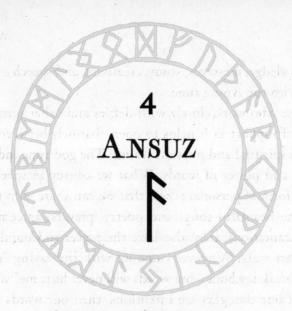

4

ANSUZ

ᚠ

Phonetic equivalent: A
Communication, Divinity, Wisdom

Great Ansuz I do call on thee
Please share with me a sign
And whisper words of poetry
From perfect lips divine

nsuz (pronounced ahn-sooz) is the rune of intelligence and communication. It is the birth of consciousness that follows the event
of cosmic creation. The Proto-Germanic translation of *Ansuz* is "god,"
and the rune is directly connected with the Norse god Odin, who is
famous for making incredible sacrifices in the pursuit of wisdom and
knowledge. In one of his better-known myths, Odin sacrifices himself *to himself* by piercing his torso with a spear and hanging from the
World Tree, which then became known as the Yggdrasil, or Odin's
Horse. He hung for nine days and nights in exchange for the divine
knowledge of the runes. In another myth, Odin gives up one of his
eyes for a drink from the well of Mímir, which is filled with the waters
of infinite wisdom.

Odin, who also goes by the names of Woden or Wodenaz, is
the root of the English word *Wednesday* (Woden's day). In terms of
magickal energy, Wednesdays support workings of communication,

gaining knowledge, messages, study, creativity, and speech—all things associated with the Ansuz rune.

For those who work closely with deities and other spirits, Ansuz is a source of support as it helps to open channels between two parties, both in spiritual and physical realms. The god rune indicates the importance and power of words. What we convey in speech and in writing is a form of personal power that we can share with the world. Words create beautiful songs and poetry, prayers, agreements, and magickal incantations; they also have the power to wound, manipulate, and start wars. Whoever came up with the saying "sticks and stones may break my bones, but words will never hurt me" was terribly mistaken. If our thoughts are intentions, then our words are spells, and they are ingrained with power. Ansuz reminds us of this power we possess and warns us to use it wisely. The well-known *Abracadabra* is the perfect example of this. It is believed that the magickal word is rooted in Aramaic and translates to "I create with words."

In readings, Ansuz may indicate an incoming message and the need to be receptive. If the reading focuses on relationships or other social matters, communication is being highlighted. For inquiries regarding one's practice, Ansuz may highlight the practitioner's relationships to the ancestors, spirits, or deities. With Kenaz, Ansuz may be expressing that an obscure message is waiting to be deciphered. Paired with Ehwaz, communication between romantic partners is the likely subject. With Ehwaz it may also suggest an animal who's reaching out and trying to get your attention. Reason, creativity (especially of the written or spoken kind), and the life force (which is called *ond* in Icelandic or *prana* in Sanskrit) are additional meanings. The ond is the life-giving breath that Odin gifted the first humans, Embla and Aske, whom he created from trees. The breath, which gives us life, simultaneously provides a means of expression through words and creativity as we string words together in the form of song and poetry.

Magickally, Ansuz is an ally for those who wish to build relationships with the divine or increase wisdom and esoteric knowledge. This rune assists poets and writers in their work and strengthens the voices of those who struggle to speak their truth. In yet another myth, Odin cleverly steals the mead of poetry called Óðrœrir, which translates to "stirrer of inspiration" in old Norse. The mead, which was made from the blood of a very wise man, held the power to endow poetic genius to anyone who drank of it. After stealing the Óðrœrir, Odin transforms into an eagle and flies away to Asgard with the mead in his beak. Before his arrival to Asgard, however, a few drops of Óðrœrir fall to the Earth, providing humanity with the gift of the creative word: *poetry*.

For creative inspiration, we can easily find a muse in nature just as we can with the Ansuz rune. Artistry is an amazing way to strengthen our bond with the Earth and merge passion with existence, whether you write, paint, dance, or play music. My creative process of choice has always been writing—poetry, short stories, prose, and I even spent a couple of years writing copy for a retail website. Sometimes I'm in the mood to write, but my "creative flow" feels blocked. Not many things can clear this sort of blockage quite like the fresh air and natural surroundings of the great outdoors. Sometimes just being outside, whether in secluded nature or a busy park, is enough to get my wheels turning again. Not only does immersing myself in the outdoors help to uncloud my mind, it also inevitably increases my gratitude toward nature. It's a win-win. A friend of mine who is an incredible musician will trek out to the woods with his guitar in tow when he's writing new songs. While not all activities can be easily accomplished outside, being in nature prior to the activity helps to cultivate the meditative mindset needed for the creative process.

I'd be remiss if I were to discuss Ansuz rewilding techniques without touching on communication. Nature is always communicating with us, and learning to discern its messages can be a lifelong practice, particularly for those like me who aren't naturally gifted in these subtler forms of communication. It took me a long time to set aside logic and stop listening with my ears—it sounds corny to say, but you really do have to "listen" with your heart.

Before I understood the concept of communicating with the green world (and trust me, I'm still learning) I was frustrated as all hell when I'd hear other folks discussing plant communication. I remember in my very first herbalism course, the instructor suggested asking a plant's permission before harvesting it. I recall feeling quite annoyed with the statement. *What do you mean **ask** them?! They never say anything back!* I never gave up, though, and continued to search for what that meant. Something I've learned about practicing magick is that usually when we try hard, we don't get the results we want; it's when we surrender and let go of expectations that the magick happens.

So, I stopped trying so hard to *listen* and allowed myself to just sit with nature, no expectations or agendas. For me, mindfulness meditation was the key to unlocking my communication conundrum. Being present and still allowed me the chance to receive messages that normally would be overlooked—messages that might arise as sensations, impressions, or emotions. Eventually, I understood what my instructor meant when she suggested asking for permission rather than just plucking plants from the ground willy-nilly. Keep in mind that, just like people, some plants want to commune and some do not. Some will be interested in creating a bond while others will not. Those that do share an interest in forming a relationship become what are known as plant spirit familiars or plant allies, and they may assist the witch in their magick much like an animal familiar would.

If this sort of communication does not come naturally to you, know that there are others out there that share in your frustration. For some this is a natural ability, while others must learn it along their journey. The best way to access this form of subtle communication is to spend as much time with plants as possible, wild or cultivated. It's like being in a foreign country—if one remains long enough, they eventually learn the language. Hail, Ansuz!

CORRESPONDENCES OF ANSUZ

ELEMENT	Air
ZODIAC	Gemini
PLANET	Mercury
MOON PHASE	Full
TAROT	The Magician, The Heirophant
CRYSTAL	Amazonite
CHAKRA	Throat
DEITIES	Cerridwen, Hermes, Mímir, Minerva, Odin, Thoth
PLANTS	Bergamot, Clary Sage, Horehound, Rowan, Sage, Sandalwood, Spikenard, Yarrow

The herbal correspondences of Ansuz aid in strengthening communication skills, deciphering messages, attaining wisdom, and fostering otherworldly relationships. Tasseomancy (reading tea leaves as a form of divination) combines the magick of Ansuz with herbcraft and is an excellent way to discover any messages you feel are being sent your way.

Bergamot
(*Monarda didyma, Citrus bergamia*)

Bergamot resides under the rulership of the Sun, and its bright citrus-y scent helps to cut through mental fog and reveal creativity and clarity. One of its many talents includes helping one change their perspective when viewing a complicated situation through a particularly unhelpful or perhaps even harmful lens. Bergamot promotes heartfelt honesty and works well for spells and rituals aimed at strengthening romantic relationships and increasing healthy communication. The uplifting citrus scent can also aid in developing psychic abilities and teaching one to trust their own intuition. Bergamot is great for restoring a sense of balance and autonomy in one's magickal practice and life.

Medicinal Properties

Bergamot's fresh citrus scent is a staple in fragrances, teas, and aroma-therapy. It is one of the main ingredients in the popular Earl Grey tea. The essential oil targets and relieves tension, soothes colic, treats gastric issues, and alleviates menstrual cramps. Sweet and bitter scents such as bergamot and grapefruit help to subdue sugar and alcohol cravings, and as someone with a hefty sweet tooth, I can certainly attest to this! Actions: analgesic, antibacterial, antifungal, anti-inflammatory, anti-spasmodic, aromatic, diuretic, expectorant, febrifuge, laxative, relaxant, stimulant. Neutral.

Clary Sage
(*Salvia sclarea*)

When it feels like your head is unorganized and full of fog, the essential oil or incense of clary sage is a cleansing and clarifying remedy. It's one of my go-to oils when preparing blends meant to stimulate mental and psychic abilities. This member of the mint family is a great choice when one's judgment is clouded, aiding in objectivity and the ability to make wise decisions. It can enhance vision in both the physical eyes and the "mind's eye" and promote calming, deep meditation or trance states. Clary sage aids in divination and visionary work of any kind. When clarity of mind and divine connection are desired, trace Ansuz between the brows with a clary sage oil blend and feel your third eye opening.

Medicinal Properties

The scent of clary sage is uplifting and calming. The essential oil is an ally for soothing stress, anxiety, and grief. It helps to dispel worry and boosts energy levels, especially if low energy is the result of anxiety and/or sadness. Clary sage benefits digestion, improves memory, soothes menstrual cramps, and relieves menopause symptoms. Traditionally it has been used as a compress for ailments of the eyes. Actions: antiseptic, antispasmodic, aperitive, aromatic, astringent, carminative, estrogenic, hypotensive, nervine, pectoral, stomachic, tonic. Avoid internal use. Cooling and balancing. Avoid during pregnancy.

Horehound
(*Marrubium vulgare*)

Horehound was once referred to as "seed of Horus" by the ancient Egyptians. Not only is it sacred to the god Horus but also to his parents, Osiris and Isis. Bathing in or drinking this mercurial herb as tea helps to cleanse and purify one's aura while dissolving creative blocks, improving cognitive function, and heightening intuition. Working with horehound in these ways is beneficial prior to divination or banishing magick. It lends power to spiritual and psychic healing, as well as home blessings. Horehound is a visionary herb that prepares the mind and spirit for traveling through liminal spaces.

Medicinal Properties

Horehound benefits myriad respiratory complaints including wheezing, asthma, bronchitis, and tuberculosis. It is often found as an ingredient in lozenges and cough syrups. As a gargle, it helps to relieve the pain of a sore throat or toothache. Horehound stimulates appetite and digestion and relieves dyspepsia, bloating, and diarrhea. It works well to treat type 2 diabetes by lowering blood sugar levels. As an anti-inflammatory, it aids in relieving spasms and cramps and is especially helpful for menstrual pain. Actions: anti-arrhythmic, astringent, bitter, cardiac, decongestant, diaphoretic, digestive, expectorant, laxative, pectoral, vermifuge. Cooling and drying. Avoid during pregnancy.

Rowan
(*Sorbus aucuparia*)

Rowan, known as the mountain ash in the United States, is one of Europe's most revered and magickal trees. It holds a rich history of protective magick, especially against curses and malefic influence. The berries enhance communication with those in the spirit realm, namely elementals, ancestors, and astral guides. When used in a jam, the berries make a delightfully sweet offering for the otherworldly beings one wishes to interact with. Burn the dried ground berries during deity invocation or evocation. On Samhain, burning a bundle of rowan twigs helps to defend against unwanted spirits from entering one's space. Because it is a tree known for its wisdom and magick, its wood is popular for making staffs, wands, and runes. Norse lore in particular has recommended the wood for dowsing rods when searching for buried treasure.

Medicinal Properties

The antioxidant-rich berries, or pomes, of the rowan tree are best ingested as a decoction, as it's never recommended to consume the berries raw due to the toxicity of the seeds. Decoctions may be used as a gargle to soothe sore throats. Rowan berries benefit asthma, diabetes, and digestive complaints including bloating, diarrhea, and constipation. They are a source of vitamin C and fiber. Actions: antibacterial, anti-inflammatory, antiseptic, astringent, digestive, nervine, stimulant. Warming and drying.

Sage (*Salvia officinalis*)

Much like the insightful thinkers, gurus, and yogis who bear the same name, sage is a plant of deep ancient wisdom. A member of the mint family, it promotes clarity, grounding, and skilled judgment. Since antiquity sage has been valued as a true healer and energetic cleanser. It is a seeker of truth and builder of emotional fortitude. It works to integrate the knowledge gained from past experience with the present, resulting in healthy judgment and decision-making. Those looking to strengthen their intuition will find an ally in sage, which also seeks to calm an overactive mind. Sage has long been sacred to Native Americans and used for its abilities to purify and drive away harmful energies.

Medicinal Properties

Sage's Latin name, *Salvia,* means "to cure or save." An Italian proverb speaks of its talent as an herb of longevity stating, "Why should a man die when sage is in his garden?" This hardy aromatic perennial works to enhance the memory, regulate menstruation, and boost digestion. It is an ally for those with menopause as it effectively decreases hot flashes and fights osteoporosis. Apply sage as a poultice for bug bites and stings. As an infusion it may be gargled to alleviate a sore throat. Fresh leaves may be chewed to strengthen the gums. Sage is a natural food preservative due to its antibacterial properties. Its astringent properties help to prevent the overproduction of sebum, which can result in overly oily skin and hair. Actions: antibacterial, anti-inflammatory, antioxidant, antiseptic, antispasmodic, astringent, digestive, diuretic, estrogenic, expectorant, styptic. Warming and drying. Those with epilepsy should avoid the essential oil. Use of the essential oil in general should be limited. Those who are breastfeeding should use with caution.

Sandalwood
(*Santalum album*)

Sandalwood is the sacred resin of the Indian sandalwood tree, valued for its high vibrational qualities. For millennia it's been praised for its abilities of purification, protection, invocation, meditation, exorcism, and astral travel. The fragrant smoke clears auric buildup and psychic channels to help better engage with the divine. Sandalwood may be burned to cleanse a space or applied as an anointing oil for the body and any tools used in ritual. Prior to meditation anoint the self with sandalwood oil, assume a favorite meditation posture, take a few deep breaths, and intone "Ansuz" until the desired state of relaxation or even trance has been achieved. Once in a calm, receptive state, you may begin to call on a choice deity or energy. When working with entities it is important to give offerings, and sandalwood incense is perfect for just that.

Medicinal Properties
In ayurvedic medicine, sandalwood has a history of treating sexually transmitted diseases (particularly gonorrhea), bronchitis, and abdominal or chest pain. While its effects are calming, it also works to stimulate cognitive function. It helps to manage symptoms of the common cold, indigestion, and urinary complaints. Sandalwood treats various skin ailments such as herpes, dermatitis, MRSA, and may even help prevent skin cancer. Unfortunately, it is at risk for overharvesting in parts of the globe, so be sure to source responsibly. Actions: anti-inflammatory, antiseptic, anxiolytic, aromatic, carminative, diuretic, stimulant, stomachic, vulnerary. Warming.

Spikenard
(*Aralia racemosa*)

Spikenard, or *nard-dog* as I like to call it (*The Office,* anyone?) is the student's herb, and for thousands of years it has been used to help with focus, retainment of information, and mental clarity. It aids the student in the comprehension of complex subject matter, whether magickal or mundane. As a tonic, spikenard may be ingested prior to learning and used as an incense during study. This perennial herb is most helpful when attaining occult knowledge through research, magick, or while working with Ansuz itself. As an herb of love, spikenard encourages healthy communication between partners as well as fidelity.

Medicinal Properties

Spikenard essential oil is a staple in aromatherapy due to its uplifting aroma. Medicinally, it is best known for its effectiveness in treating asthma, colds, and general cough. It helps to clear the lungs after quitting smoking. Spikenard is ideal for skin conditions including dandruff, eczema, psoriasis, and those of the fungal variety, namely athlete's foot. It works to purify the blood. Actions: antibacterial, alterative, antifungal, anti-inflammatory, antirheumatic, carminative, diaphoretic, diuretic, expectorant, stimulant. Warming and drying. Avoid during pregnancy.

Yarrow
(*Achillea millefolium*)

Yarrow's Latin name derives from Achilles, an ancient Greek warrior who treasured the plant for its abilities to treat battle wounds and clot bleeding. Along with Achilles, it's associated with Aphrodite, Cernunnos, and Chiron the centaur. The stocks are commonly used in the Chinese divination system of I Ching. Because of its ability to bring about knowledge and clarity, yarrow is a popular herb in all forms of divination. To increase psychic ability, burn as incense, add to a ritual bath, or create an infused oil for predivination use. This North American native stimulates creative energies and inspiration. Yarrow not only heals physical injury but also works well for the healing of emotional wounds. It is an excellent ally for those who suffer from chronic depression, as it encourages confidence, hope, and an optimistic outlook. Place beneath a pillow to induce prophetic dreaming. As an herb of Venus, yarrow is often associated with love, especially healthy communication among lovers. Hang over a couple's shared bed or keep some under the mattress to promote clear communication and a happy relationship.

Medicinal Properties

Among its many talents, yarrow is first and foremost a prized wound healer. It is strongly styptic and antiseptic. In the event of a large wound, it may be applied to staunch the bleeding until the appropriate medical care is available. Yarrow remedies fevers, high blood pressure, heavy menstrual bleeding and cramping, and seasonal allergies. It targets pain, particularly toothaches and headaches. *Encyclopedia of Herbal Medicine* by Andrew Chevallier recommends an infusion of equal parts yarrow, peppermint, and elder flower for colds, which can be taken three times daily while symptoms persist. An infusion may be used as a wash for irritated eyes.* Yarrow is beneficial to the overall health of the liver and kidneys. Actions: anti-inflammatory, antiseptic, antispasmodic, antiviral, astringent, bitter tonic, diaphoretic, diuretic, febrifuge, hemostatic, styptic, vulnerary. Cooling and drying. Not for long-term use. Toxic to dogs and cats. Avoid during pregnancy and nursing.

---

*Andrew Chevallier, *Encyclopedia of Herbal Medicine* (London, England: Penguin Random House, 2016), 56.

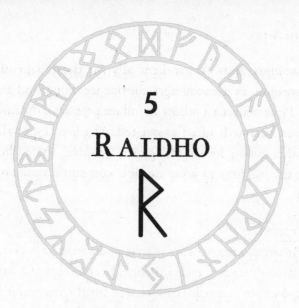

5
RAIDHO

Phonetic equivalent: R
Travel, Journey, Decisions

Raidho is my heart
Every step is a beat
Each path that I wander
Is kissed by my feet

Raidho (pronounced rye-tho) is the travel rune—the name itself translates to "riding" in Proto-Germanic. It represents journey, movement, control, and curiosity. It is within our very natures to wonder and wander, to question and explore. Humans travel for many reasons today, and perhaps mostly to experience cultures and landscapes foreign from one's own. It's how we learn, remain humble, and see the grander scheme of things far beyond our front doors.

In ancient times, traveling was done by foot, boat, and horse. The Norwegian rune poem calls riding "worst for horses," suggesting the physical stress that riding puts on the animal. Today the terms *travel* and *journey* conjure images of airplanes, trains, motor vehicles, and boats. Some prefer to travel by foot, backpacking over large distances. There's an entire underground movement of homeless-by-choice train-riding transients who live off odd jobs, seasonal farm work, and panhandling, some of whom I've met with Raidho tattoos.

Not only does Raidho represent the act of travel but also the paths on which we do so. Life itself is the ultimate journey, and each individual's path is paved with decisions. Many, like me, prefer to think that humans have the freedom of choice, that our fates are not sealed as soon as we exit the womb. Our "nows" are direct results of the choices we've previously made. Mistakes are an inevitable part of everyone's journey—we all take wrong turns and get tripped up on our paths from time to time. Such mistakes serve to teach and fortify us. Along the road, we become better navigators, callouses build on our feet to protect them from the rough pavement below, and we learn to detect storms before they strike—this is the metaphorical path of wisdom. When we stop and look over our own life's path, we can see how the concept of choice is closely tied to the Raidho rune. Within spiritual communities, we often hear phrases like, "path to enlightenment," "astral travel," or "spiritual quest." These phrases help to illustrate clear timelines of goal attainment and inner growth. On the spirit level, Raidho is a wonderful ally for those who traverse the boundaries that separate the physical and otherworldly realms—the shamans, hedge witches, and völvas (A Norse seeress). The nine worlds of the Yggdrasil tree stands as the axis mundi within spirit travel and can serve as a map for such travels.

In a reading Raidho may be foretelling that a journey is in the near future, whether in the spiritual or physical sense. On a psychological level, it can represent leadership, choice, and the ability to control a situation versus being controlled *by* it. The appearance of this rune may be asking you to consider your choices and the current direction you're going. Is it time to change direction? Raidho paired with Isa may warn against moving too fast or overworking and indicate the need to slow down or even come to a full stop. Alongside Jera, the message may be to keep up the momentum.

Reversed or murkstave, Raidho can represent problematic choices, a fruitless voyage, or a warning to hold off on a planned journey. In the spiritual sense it could point to stagnation, the inability to make decisions, losing control, or feeling lost on your life journey. Agoraphobia and xenophobia are extreme examples of reversed Raidho.

Wouldn't it be grand to quit your job and travel the world to climb mountains, sail seas, trek through deserts, and hike rainforests? I think so, but for most of us it's not going to happen for reasons such as jobs, finances, family, or limitations in physical ability. Jetting around the globe is definitely a romantic way to strengthen the Earth bond, but traveling for pleasure is a luxury that not everyone has. For some, even getting out into nature regularly is not a possibility, especially those who reside in cities. So how do we get our fix? One way is through inner journeying. Inner journeying is done through methods of visualization, trance, and even astral projection. It's not unheard of for all three to occur in one sitting. Over the years I have created for myself an *inner landscape*—a concept introduced to me by my first herbalism instructor, and the practice has literally opened up a new world to me. It is a familiar spot I can return to anytime—one filled with a thick, verdant forest, plant and animal allies, and of course, magick.

I begin the process of inner journeying alone in a quiet room; preferably dark as well. If it's light outside, I'll wear a sleep mask or drape a dark shawl over my eyes. If it's nighttime, I will turn off all lights and light one single candle that will serve as my focal point to help shift my consciousness. This is the best time to employ any relaxation methods, such as deep breathing techniques or playing or listening to percussive music to prepare the mind for inner journeying.

When you feel completely grounded and centered, focus. Activate your mind's eye and see yourself alone in a void. Nothing exists around you; there is no north, south, east, or west. After a short time of experiencing quiet nothingness, you suddenly see what appears to be a small door off in the distance. As you approach it you see that it is in fact an old, weathered door. It is inviting amid the nothingness. Reach in your pocket and pull out an antique skeleton key. Feel it in your hand before sliding it into the keyhole. Once the door is unlocked, open it, step inside, and close the door behind you.

You have just entered your outdoor sanctuary. You have a blank canvas to make this place whatever you want. What do you see when you first enter? Is it night or day? Are there animals around? What kind of plants adorn your space? Bit by bit, create your sanctuary. Spare no details. Take your time with it. This is where you can get deep into nature without even leaving your home.

When I first step through my door, I am greeted by clusters of elder trees and other plant allies of mine like mugwort, mullein, and vervain. In the center of the trees is a raging bonfire. It's perpetual nighttime and the moon is bright and full. The stars look like silver glitter on an endless stretch of the deepest blue. There are unlit candles and lanterns all around, and in this place I have the ability to ignite their flames with a mere point of my finger.

I am barefoot and do my best to "feel" the cool soil and grass beneath my feet as I move about. My cats, Franny and Dee, who passed away a few years back, live there and they are living their best lives. They playfully chase each other and other critters, they eat all the tuna and yogurt their hearts desire, and they love curling up together near the ever-burning fire. There is plentiful wildlife in my space, fireflies, moss-covered boulders, and gorgeous colonies of fungi.

Not far beyond the grove of hawthorn trees is a stream and a single towering weeping willow tree. Like all the plants and animals in my landscape, the willow is a close ally, but this tree in particular has a special purpose—if and when I decide to venture beyond the safety of my landscape, I begin my journey beneath the willow, where I'm enveloped in an undulating sphere of protective golden light. Once I am shielded, I thank the tree, leave an offering, and cross the stream via a small rustic bridge made entirely of unaltered tree branches. About twenty yards ahead of me is the tree line of an endless forest. This tree line is the boundary between sanctuary (conscious) and unknown (sub- or unconscious). This is normally about the time where voluntary visualization ends and deep trance takes over.

Once I enter the forest, I am in strange territory, no matter how many times I've traveled it. It is ever-changing. It is in this forest that I met my animal guide, a sometimes grumpy but otherwise lovable elderly wolf. I never know what I will encounter when I enter the woods. Sometimes my guide accompanies me, and other times he lets me know that I must go it alone. Every now and again I find myself in frightening situations, confronted by ill-intentioned entities, hiking treacherous terrain, or caught in a raging storm. Just as in real life, the difficulties that I face here often yield lessons and bits of wisdom applicable to the current happenings of my life.

When I am ready to leave the forest, I make my way back toward my sanctuary (consciousness). I always intuitively know how to return no matter how far off the beaten path I've wandered. It is a place where I am always safe; a place where harmful entities and energies cannot exist. Sometimes I stay for long periods of time, cuddling my kitties, exchanging energy with my plant allies, and meditating by the fire. And sometimes I quickly say my good-byes, step through the rickety wooden door, and lock it behind me knowing that I will return soon.

I invite you to map out and build your inner landscape. Even if you prefer not to venture beyond the confines of your safe zone, you still have your own personal piece of unadulterated wilderness where you can retreat and meditate whenever the mood strikes. Hail, Raidho!

CORRESPONDENCES OF RAIDHO

ELEMENT	Earth
ZODIAC	Sagittarius
PLANET	Jupiter
MOON PHASE	New Moon
TAROT	The Chariot
CRYSTAL	Moonstone
CHAKRA	Solar Plexus
DEITIES	Abeona/Adiona, Ganesha, Khonsu, Mercury, Odin, Yacatecuhtli
PLANTS	Ash, Calamus, Comfrey, Datura, Feverfew, Mugwort, Thyme

The corresponding plants of Raidho offer protection and guidance to the travelers of physical journeys as well as those navigating travels of spiritual nature. They work to help the practitioner take charge of their destiny and cultivate authentic living.

Ash
(*Fraxinus excelsior*)

In Norse mythology, the god Odin transforms two trees into the first humans: Embla from an elm and Aske from an ash tree. Ash, a tree in the olive family, is argued to be the mighty Yggdrasil, although some believe it to be yew. This flowering tree has a long esoteric history and variety of magickal uses, which include protection from drowning, removal of warts, divination, sea rituals, lucid dreaming, and more. The leaves may be used to bring travelers safely home, and because of the associations to Water and Neptune, ash is especially beneficial for those traveling by water. For a quick and easy travel safety charm, inscribe Raidho on an ash leaf and keep it in your vehicle or in a travel bag. Because of its inclusion in Norse myth and Druid history, the wood of the tree is perfect for rune and staff making; if possible take wood from a branch that has already fallen. If one should decide to cut a branch from the tree, be sure to ask permission first and leave an offering in return.

Medicinal Properties
Ash is rarely used in modern plant medicine. Historically, the bark and leaves were used as remedies for fevers, constipation, and jaundice. A poultice of the leaves may be applied to the skin to soothe bug bites. As a diuretic it helps relieve and prevent kidney stones and urinary tract infections. Actions: astringent, bitter tonic, diaphoretic, diuretic, hepatic, laxative.

Calamus
(*Acorus calamus*)

In magick, calamus is associated with control. While Raidho is thought of mainly as the travel rune, it is also the rune associated with control, decisions, and taking charge of one's destiny. Within hoodoo, calamus is often used to exert influence or control and is a main ingredient in *commanding powder,* which gives the user the upper hand over whomever they choose. Because of its impressive powers of persuasion, this aromatic plant is frequently included in love spells and baneful magick.

It may be applied to protection, purification, sanctification, and is commonly added to sacred incense blends. To ensure that you remain the one in control during spirit communication, burn a calamus and frankincense blend while invoking the commanding powers of Raidho.

Medicinal Properties

Calamus, also known as sweet flag, is valued for its strongly medicinal rhizomes. It is widely used within ayurvedic medicine for its digestive benefits. Taken as an infusion or decoction, calamus helps increase appetite. It is revitalizing to the nervous system. The essential oil is toxic in large amounts, but in small amounts it has myriad benefits such as memory enhancement, relief from insomnia, improved circulation, and arthritis relief. Actions: anti-inflammatory, antioxidant, antispasmodic, aphrodisiac, aromatic, bitter, carminative, emetic, nervine, stimulant, vulnerary. Slightly warming. Avoid calamus during pregnancy and nursing. Avoid alongside heart disorders.

Comfrey
(*Symphytum officinale*)

Like Raidho, comfrey is an agent of travel. It has been used as a safety charm since antiquity, providing the traveler with protection from injury, illness, thieves, and general misfortune while ensuring a safe return. Before embarking on a journey, sprinkle comfrey and mugwort in shoes, luggage, or vehicle. If checking bags on a flight or bus, the wanderer's herb will aid in the prevention of lost luggage. To create a protective amulet for your vehicle, place a few pinches of comfrey and other travel herbs in a small pouch, include a bindrune of Raidho, Elhaz, and Ehwaz, and hang it from your rearview mirror. Just be sure it won't obstruct your vision, as that would be quite counterproductive as a safety charm! Comfrey aids in providing the courage and assertiveness necessary to set healthy boundaries as well as the wisdom to know when it's time to let go of someone or something. For those in need of quick healing, especially from broken bones, a bundle of the dried herb should be kept near the bed. Grow it near the entrances of home to ward off people or spirits with ill intentions. Due to its Earth element correspondence, comfrey is an ideal choice for helping one achieve grounding.

Medicinal Properties

Comfrey possesses the amazing ability to proliferate cells and is a very useful topical remedy. It benefits various skin conditions including acne, cuts and scrapes, fungal infections, and rashes. Because it works so well at sealing the top layer of skin, it should never be used for deep punctures or lacerations as it can potentially seal in bacteria. When applied as a poultice it encourages the healing of broken bones, sprains, and fractures. Because of such qualities, comfrey has been used to treat the mosquito-borne disease dengue fever, which often results in joint pain. In eastern Europe, a decoction of the root is served as a traditional remedy for dry cough. Comfrey relieves diarrhea when taken internally; however, it's recommended that you work with a healthcare professional regarding dosage. Actions: alterative, analgesic, astringent, demulcent, emollient, expectorant, nutritive, refrigerant, styptic, vulnerary. Cooling and moistening. Avoid during pregnancy and nursing.

Datura
(*Datura stramonium*)

Datura has a history of aiding in spirit travel among shamans. It helps to guide and protect those who journey beyond the physical world. Traditionally, its intoxicating properties have been used to aid in prophecy, spirit communication, visionary practices, and the breaking of hexes and curses. This member of the nightshade family corresponds to deities such as Kali, Nyx, Hel, Hekate, and Saturn. As a chthonic herb it helps one to reconcile their feelings and beliefs regarding death and the afterlife. Datura, also known as jimsonweed, devil's weed, and thornapple, is a poisonous plant and should only be handled with protective gear.

Medicinal Properties

Due to its toxicity, datura is not recommended for medicinal usage. Traditionally it has been used to relieve inflammation and nervous disorders. Actions: anodyne, anti-inflammatory, aphrodisiac, hallucinogenic, sedative, vulnerary. Cooling and moistening. For dosage information consult with a professional herbalist. Do not handle while pregnant or nursing.

Feverfew
(*Tanacetum parthenium*)

Feverfew is a nurturing Venusian herb that seeks to heal and protect. It is an ally for those who are accident prone and works to ensure safety, particularly during travel. Feverfew aids in mental acuity and nurtures creativity by dispelling the harmful energies that tend to cloud judgment. It intensifies healing spells and rituals, especially when illness seems to be lingering or if one falls ill while far from home. Hang dried bundles of the herb in the room of a sick individual to help attract healing energies.

Medicinal Properties

From the name, it's pretty clear what feverfew's abilities are touted for. Taken as hot tea it is an effective remedy for fevers. The name for this type of remedy is *febrifuge,* which comes from the Latin word for "fever," which is *febris.* While fevers are necessary to kill infection, those that reach dangerously high temperatures quickly become health risks and require relief. When taken regularly, feverfew helps to prevent migraine headaches, especially for those who tend to get them in clusters or during menstruation. I am a sufferer of cluster migraines, and I use a tincture of feverfew and lavender as a preventative measure. Feverfew treats chest congestion, asthma, coughs, and sore throats. Topical ointments soothe insect stings and bites. The anti-inflammatory and digestive properties of feverfew work to alleviate gastritis, especially when paired with similar herbs. Actions: analgesic, anti-inflammatory, carminative, digestive, emetic, emmenagogue, expectorant, febrifuge, nervine. Cooling and drying. Feverfew may cause allergic reaction. Avoid alongside anticoagulants and the weeks preceding a surgery. Avoid during pregnancy and nursing.

Mugwort
(*Artemisia vulgaris*)

Mugwort is a mildly psychoactive plant capable of extraordinary magick. It's truly an herb that every witch should have on hand, because not only does it help us to travel beyond the mundane, it also provides protection along the way as well. Mugwort is a guardian of mothers, children, and the process of childbirth. Its maternal nature is reflected in its moniker *Mother of Herbs* and works quite well when paired with Perthro or Berkana. For travel, it is traditionally sprinkled in the shoes or coat pocket before departure. Astral travelers will find a trusty companion in mugwort as it facilitates the necessary state of mind and helps with safe return to the body. It's a popular visionary aid and may be ingested as tea or tincture, smoked, or burned as incense before divination. It's one of my personal favorites for the making of smoke wands. To achieve lucid dreaming, sip the hot tea before bed or add a bit of mugwort and lavender inside of a pillowcase. Regarding the wheel of the year, mugwort corresponds to Samhain and is also one of the nine sacred herbs of the Anglo-Saxons. To better connect with nature, sprinkle a bit of the herb in your shoes before hiking. Not only will this encourage bonding with the fauna and flora around you, it will also provide safety along the way.

Medicinal Properties

The motherly mugwort plant is an advocate for feminine health. It helps to induce labor, birth the placenta, and relieve excessive post-partum bleeding. As a strong emmenagogue, it increases blood flow to the uterus and encourages menstruation. As a stimulant for the digestive system, it promotes a healthy appetite. Bathe in mugwort to soothe sore muscles or general skin irritations including poison ivy, oak, and sumac. Drinking the hot tea induces sweating and relieves high fevers while supporting uterine health. Actions: analgesic, anti-bacterial, antifungal, anti-inflammatory, antirheumatic, aromatic, astringent, bitter, carminative, cholagogue, choleretic, diaphoretic, emmenagogue, expectorant, nervine, uterine stimulant, vermifuge. Warming and drying. While Mugwort is ideal for bringing on labor, avoid over the course of pregnancy due to its uterine stimulating actions. Avoid while nursing.

Thyme
(*Thymus vulgaris*)

Thyme may seem like an unassuming culinary herb, but along with its aromatic and flavorful abilities it is actually quite the visionary aid and is often paired with divination or astral travel. It helps to provide the ethereal traveler with a cloak of power and protection. Over the centuries, thyme has been used as a general energy cleanser and booster of magick while simultaneously driving away malicious spirits (and mosquitos, too!) when burned. Thyme is quite lighthearted, but stern when it needs to be. It provides courage when it is needed. For those who work with the fae, this invigorating herb makes for an excellent offering. During Samhain when the veil is at its thinnest, add thyme to the sabbat dinner to invite passed loved ones to the table; and be sure to offer them their own plates. Drink as a tea or add it to a ritual bath to promote confidence and bravery before journeying to other realms. Add thyme to baths to cleanse the aura and fill it with ebullient energy.

Medicinal Properties

Thyme is an aromatic herb that targets lung infections like bronchitis and whooping cough. It contains antioxidants that help counter the effects of aging. Thyme helps to treat and prevent stomach ulcers. It may be taken as tea, tincture, or supplement for asthma and seasonal allergies. The strong antifungal properties treat infections such as ringworm, athlete's foot, and thrush. Its antiparasitic qualities are effective against lice and scabies. The tea may be used as a mouthwash for toothaches, cavities, and gingivitis. Thyme helps to prevent and treat epileptic seizures. Using the tincture externally on acne dries breakouts. Actions: antifungal, antioxidant, antiseptic, antispasmodic, aromatic, antiviral, bronchodilator, carminative, emmenagogue, expectorant, vermifuge. Warming and drying. Avoid the essential oil while pregnant or breastfeeding. Avoid before surgery.

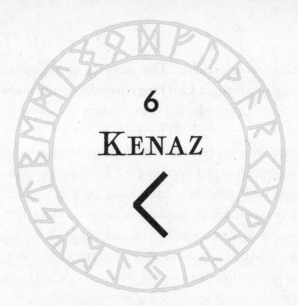

6
KENAZ

Phonetic equivalent: K and hard C
Torch, Heat, Passion

The Kenaz torch shines its light about
The deep forest as I journey throughout
It wraps me in warmth on the coldest of nights
A flame roaring inside of me, a beacon so bright

Kenaz (pronounced kay-nahz) translates to "beacon" or "torch" in Proto-Germanic and is a symbol of illumination, heat, transformation, craft, and knowledge. Its meaning is reflected in the shape of the stave, which resembles rays of light shining outward from a single source.

Kenaz is passion, sexuality, and creativity. It's what gives us drive and purpose. The Norwegian and Icelandic rune poems refer to the rune as a "blister" or "sore" indicating the outcome of making contact with extreme heat and suggesting the need to take care when working with the torch rune.

The torch has always been symbolic for finding one's way through the metaphorical dark, and Kenaz can be a great ally for those courageous enough to explore it. Psychologically, this darkness is the deep psyche of the human mind. Hidden away from the light are repressed memories, urges, feelings, and thoughts. The unconscious contains all that we consider unacceptable about ourselves. This grouping of hidden characteristics is what famed psychologist Carl Jung referred to as the shadow. Jung's theories have been largely adopted into modern occultism due to his research involving dreams, symbols, theology, archetypes, and more. Jung theorized that we hide our flaws and maladaptive tendencies in order to feel better about ourselves and possibly even feel superior to others. The theory also explains that while we think we are tucking our shadows away, they contribute widely to our daily behaviors and thought patterns and manifest in our dreams, typically to our dismay.

Today, the introspective practice of shadow work is gaining traction, particularly within spiritual and occult communities. It is considered a way to seek out and reconcile the parts of ourselves that we've tucked away in order to heal and grow. Shadow work has been a large part of my practice and overall healing process and it's something we'll touch on a bit more in the Berkana chapter. The torch rune aids in spiritual alchemy as it guides us through the dark depths of our psyches and shines light upon the things that cause pain and dysfunction. It also provides us with the flames of transformation to alchemize undesirable traits into strengths. Simply calling upon the rune for assistance is one way to employ it while engaging in such gritty work. This may be done by enclosing yourself in a dark, quiet room and lighting one single candle into which you've carved the Kenaz stave. The candle flame will serve as an offering as well as your focal point. Assume a meditative position and keep your gaze fixed on the flame. Take a few deep breaths and intone "Kenaz" nine times (the sacred number of Norse mythology). Call out to the spirit of Kenaz and request its guidance and protection while you journey to the abandoned depths of your soul. This communication can be accomplished silently or spoken out loud, whatever you're comfortable with. Ask the spirit of the rune to accept your offering. Continue to meditate and focus on the flame until you feel centered and grounded. Once you are, shadow work can begin. Just as there are endless ways to perform a ritual, there are endless ways to work with the shadow. I recommend further study for those seriously interested in doing this type of work. As mentioned previously, there are a couple examples in the Berkana chapter.

Not only is Kenaz arguably the most beneficial rune to apply to shadow work (alongside Hagalaz and Nauthiz), it's also tremendously beneficial to the artist as it represents the initial passion that precedes the creation. It fuels the fire, so to speak. The arts are a true gift of humanity, as artistic expression allows us to channel deep emotions and apply them to the creation of beauty for beauty's sake. It's no wonder the rune that assists us in psychological exploration is also the very rune that catalyzes our artistic endeavors. Kenaz is energetic and inspiring. It promotes open-mindedness and is a reminder to question the things we are fed as factual and to seek out our own truths. Kenaz represents the acquisition of knowledge, specifically knowledge of a spiritual nature.

Within a reading, the presence of the torch rune may shine a light on information that is being overlooked or ignored. If the inquiry is about romance, Kenaz may be implying sexuality and lust. When paired with Fehu it may indicate an innovative endeavor. Reversed, Kenaz is emotional or physical burnout, boredom, a spiritual void, getting "burned" by someone, lack of creativity, psychological unrest, or ignorance. It is denial of truth and a feeling of being lost or "left in the dark." In the reversed position, Kenaz may also indicate depression, blocked creativity, over-influence of the shadow, or a loss of passion.

Kenaz encourages a connection to nature via one of its more destructive processes: fire. As it destroys, fire transforms and purifies and was therefore an attractive method of extermination in the aptly named "burning times." Scholars estimate that around fifty thousand people were executed, most of them burned at the stake under the accusations of witchcraft. The burning of bodies and leftover bones has long been used as a means of dispelling evil spirits and is the root of the term *bonfire,* or "bone fire."

Because of its ability to purify via transformation, fire is an excellent consecrator. Purification through fire is central to the practice of alchemy, especially in the making of spagyric tinctures. *Solve et coagula.* Fire is unique in that it is the only of the four elements that can be created and the only that can be extinguished by the remaining elements.

There is more to fire than its physicality. Fire is passion, rage, and lust. In its spiritual aspect it is the animator of all life. It is what moves messages through the brain and keeps the heart beating. When we die, it is said that our metaphorical "flame goes out" and our once warm and mobile bodies become cool and still.

Of course, fire does not only destroy; it provides light, warmth, and a means of preparing food. Fire was crucial to the survival of humans before gas and electricity warmed our homes and cooked our meals. Like all of the elements, it is essential and important to witchcraft Fire lights our candles, dances within our cauldrons, ignites incense, conjures, destroys, consecrates, and more. Candle magick is a simple yet effective way to call on the power of fire for spells and rituals.

The following is an effortless and quick devotional ritual to nurture the bond between nature and human. It is best done outside, but of course make do with what you've got. What you'll need:

One small green, brown, or white candle
Candleholder
A carving tool
A lighter or matches

With a sharp tool, carve a bindrune of Kenaz and Berkana into the wax of the candle. As you do so, visualize the bindrune infusing and glowing with the Fire power of Kenaz and the Earth power of Berkana. When the bindrune is complete place the candle in a holder and light the wick. Assume a meditative position such as tree pose, sitting cross-legged, or standing up straight. Breathe mindfully until a state of relaxation is achieved and you feel grounded. When ready, state a version of the following while keeping your relaxed gaze on the candle:

> *With this flickering flame*
> *I pay reverence to the Earth*
> *For it mothers all of life*
> *The source of passion, heat, and mirth*
> *Mighty Kenaz and Berkana*
> *Keep our kinship burning bright*
> *And may I always be an ally*
> *Guided by your endless light*

Close your eyes and keep the image of the candle burning bright in your mind. Remain in quiet reflection until you feel satisfied to close the ritual. Hail, Kenaz!

CORRESPONDENCES OF KENAZ

ELEMENT	Fire
ZODIAC	Leo
PLANET	Mars
MOON PHASE	New Moon
TAROT	Ace of Wands
CRYSTAL	Carnelian
CHAKRA	Sacral
DEITIES	Agneya, Hekate, Hestia, Loki, Pele, Zhurong
PLANTS	Basil, Clove, Damiana, Elecampane, Hibiscus, Kava Kava, Mullein, Yerba Santa

Similar to the herbs of Raidho, many of the corresponding herbs of Kenaz provide guidance and protection to travelers of the astral realms. The plants of Kenaz are perfect in workings of creativity, passion, love, and sex.

Basil
(*Ocimum basilicum*)

Basil is a common kitchen herb, but its talents reach far beyond its ability to flavor dishes. Like the Kenaz rune, this freshly scented herb is ruled by the element of Fire and corresponds to the planet Mars and the Norse god Tyr. Basil is magickally inclined toward workings of love, courage, protection, banishings, home cleansings, money magick, and more. During the cold months or a generally stagnant time in one's life, it may be used to strengthen one's inner fire, which can be accomplished in a variety of ways: burn as incense while meditating on the power of Kenaz, add some to a ceremonial herbal bath or hot tea blend to purify and reset energies, or keep some in a pocket or sachet when in need of courage and/or vitality. Basil may be included in formulations for banishing and exorcism. Lore points out basil's aggressively protective qualities through its connections to fearsome fiery beasts such as dragons, basilisks, and scorpions.

Medicinal Properties

Basil is a sweetly scented aromatic herb packed with antioxidants. It is a common remedy for minor skin irritations, relieving gas, easing nausea, and increasing the production of breastmilk. Its emmenagogic properties facilitate a stubborn menstrual cycle and promote the birthing of placenta after labor. Basil supports cardiovascular, gut, and liver health. It has been used as an alternative for antibiotics. Actions: antidepressant, anti-inflammatory, antioxidant, antiseptic, carminative, diaphoretic, digestive, emmenagogue, expectorant, febrifuge, nervine, stimulant, sedative, vermifuge. Warming. Avoid the essential oil during pregnancy.

Clove
(*Syzygium aromaticum*)

The scent of clove is energizing and warm, encouraging of optimism and passion. Such favorable energies aid in the healing of relationships (friend, romantic, or familial), increased sexual desire, and boosting confidence. These aromatic flower buds promote confidence and courage. Clove incense discourages jealousy and gossip while fostering healthy interactions with others—especially those you might find *challenging*. Meditating or simply being still among the heady smoke or essential oil helps prepare one for the important occasions of their life. Clove is a visionary herb with a warm, spicy flavor suitable for pre-ritual teas and elixirs. Before traveling the astral realms, prepare a hot cup of clove tea. While drinking, visualize the purifying and protective fires of Kenaz surrounding you and fortifying you in preparation for your journey.

Medicinal Properties

Clove has natural numbing qualities that aid in the soothing of minor pains such as tooth pain. To relieve a toothache, place a whole clove between the cheek and gums beside the affected tooth. Clove eases digestive upset, specifically hiccups, nausea, bloating, cramping, and gas. It aids in the restoration of lost appetite and is suitable for treating individuals who suffer from anorexia or bulimia. In aromatherapy, it is used to strengthen the memory. Actions: analgesic, antiemetic, antiseptic, antispasmodic, aromatic, carminative, counterirritant, diuretic, stimulant, vermifuge. Warming and drying. Ingesting in large amounts may cause irritation.

Damiana
(*Turnera aphrodisiaca*)

Kenaz + damiana = *bow chicka wow-wow!* Damiana, a member of the passionflower family, is one of my go-to herbal aphrodisiacs. In both magick and medicine it is a helpful aid for those working to improve their sex lives. It is often consumed to increase one's libido, especially if low sex drive is a result of depression or anxiety. It may be taken as hot tea, smoked, added to baths, added to spell bottles and sachets, or burned as incense. Personally, my favorite way to invoke damiana's lusty properties is as a powdered additive in massage oils. Pair with rose petals to create a sensual bath. A relationship with this flowering evergreen is beneficial for those who have unhealthy views about sex. This fiery herb of Scorpio is not only enjoyed for its sexual benefits but also for the enhancement of psychic abilities, which in turn aids in divination, trance work, lucid dreaming, and of course, sex magick. It helps to break down the barriers that can block one from entering and exploring the spiritual realms while providing courage for the journey itself.

Medicinal Properties

Damiana is an energizer, de-stressor, and a hormone balancer, all of which assist in increasing libido. Its nervine properties help ease anxiety, depression, and other mood disorders. It works to soothe headaches brought on by menstruation, balances blood sugar, and eases nervous stomach. Those who deal with occasional impotence may benefit from the use of damiana. It improves digestion, relieves coughs, and treats urinary tract infections. Actions: antidepressant, antiseptic, antispasmodic, aphrodisiac, diuretic, expectorant, metabolic stimulant, mild laxative, nervine, tonic. Warming. Avoid during pregnancy and nursing.

Elecampane
(*Inula helenium*)

Elecampane is also known as "elfwort" or "elf dock" due to its purported use against "elf shot"—a sudden pain that occurs from the cunning shot of an elf's arrow. It is an excellent herb to use for those who work with the fae and spirits of the land. It was valued by the Druids and ancient Celts, who used it mainly in incense form to enhance psychic abilities and dispel harmful energy. Elecampane is traditionally used for love magick and baby blessings. For the creative type, this herb is a must-have as it works to remove creative blocks and encourage fresh ideas. While burning the incense, use your finger to trace Kenaz over your third eye and envision your mental fog drifting away with the incense smoke until you feel clear-headed and ready to work!

Medicinal Properties

Elecampane is a time-tested medicine for the treatment of chronic respiratory infections, lingering wet coughs, and cleansing the lungs after one quits smoking. Its medicinal use goes all the way back to ancient Rome. The root especially is helpful as it is a strong expectorant and is also effective against diseases including tuberculosis and the antibiotic-resistant staph infection known as MRSA. Elecampane is rich in fiber, immune boosting, and strengthening to those with debility. Actions: antibacterial, antiseptic, astringent, bitter, diaphoretic, diuretic, expectorant, stimulant, vermifuge. Warming and drying. Avoid during pregnancy and nursing.

Kava Kava
(*Piper methysticum*)

Kava kava is an effective yet gentle sedative, and in magickal context it's used to relax and clear the mind for meditation and visionary work. It has mild aphrodisiacal properties and has become a staple in sex magick. In the Pacific Islands, fermented kava kava was consumed to induce altered states of consciousness for the purpose of divine communion. Call on the power of Kenaz and kava to explore sexuality—a practice that may be approached alone or with a partner. Sex and orgasm are wonderful ways to raise and harness potent energy, which may then be directed with clear intention. Not everyone is comfortable with this method of raising energy, and that's okay; to each their own. Kava has the ability to heal and soothe mild depression and is a gentle herbal aid in the healing of sexual traumas.

Medicinal Properties

Kava kava is a prized remedy for the treatment of anxiety, stress, and insomnia. It is soothing for headaches and migraines. The antiseptic and analgesic properties of kava make it useful for treating various kinds of infections, such as urinary tract infections. The tea may be used as a mouthwash for sores and tooth infections. Actions: analgesic, anesthetic, anticancer, antiseptic, antispasmodic, diuretic, sedative. Warming and drying. Kava kava is a potent sedative and muscle relaxant; one should never drink alcohol or operate a motor vehicle after consuming it. It should be avoided in extreme amounts. Avoid alongside liver disease.

Hibiscus
(*Hibiscus sabdariffa*)

Hibiscus is sacred to the Hindu deities Kali and Ganesha, to which the flowers are a perfect offering in plant or tea form. Like Kali, hibiscus is wildly passionate. It lends its powers to magick regarding love, sex, justice, confidence, and healing. Hibiscus is a freeing flower, aiding folks in the breaking of emotional bonds that keep them from moving forward. It also works to support those who have trouble expressing their sexuality. Add the dried petals to aphrodisiac incense blends, ritual baths, or love potions.

Medicinal Properties

Hibiscus is a natural hydrator and source of vitamin C. It is a valued remedy in ayurvedic medicine for anemia, hair loss, balancing hormones, increasing circulation, regulating blood pressure, and the treatment of inflammatory skin conditions. This crimson-hued flower is soothing for fevers, colds, and coughs, and promotes healthy skin and hair. Actions: antioxidant, astringent, demulcent, mild digestive, sedative. Cooling and moistening.

Mullein
(*Verbascum thapsus*)

Mullein has a long list of nicknames, some of which include candlewick plant, witches' flint, and hag's tapers. These names are a result of its large velvety leaves and their long-burning ability. Traditionally, dried leaves are cast into a ritual fire or burned as incense. To create a torch, wrap the fresh leaves around the end of a branch and allow time for the leaves to dry. Once dried, the torch may be dipped in wax and rolled into an herbal blend or ignited as is to provide just the right amount of light for nighttime rituals. The burning of mullein aids in the banishing of any harmful energies that may be in or around your space. It's a truly versatile herb ideal for love magick, protection, repelling nightmares, and safe travel, whether physical or spiritual. For travel by foot, combine with mugwort and/or comfrey and add to shoes or a vehicle charm. Mullein offers protection to those who move between realms. The powdered leaf has been used as a substitute for graveyard dirt due to its abilities to protect from evil spirits. If you can believe it, the talents of mullein even go beyond magickal and medicinal as another one of its popular nicknames is *cowboy toilet paper*. The name says it all!

Medicinal Properties

Mullein has been valued for its medicinal abilities for over two thousand years. It has an affinity for the life-giving breath and is a threat against various respiratory complaints. It may even be smoked to relieve wheezing. Use the flowers to make soothing drops for earaches that are the result of congestion. For dry cough, combine with coltsfoot to increase the remedial effectiveness. The entire plant has strong antibacterial properties. The dried root may be powdered and applied to wounds to speed up the healing process. Mullein is considered generally safe and may be used temporarily for children with ear or respiratory infections.

Actions: Leaf—alterative, anodyne, antibacterial, antihistamine, anti-inflammatory, antiseptic, antispasmodic, antiviral, astringent, decongestant, demulcent, diuretic, emollient, expectorant, pectoral, vulnerary. Flower—alterative, analgesic, antihistamine, anti-inflammatory, antispasmodic, antiviral, demulcent, emollient, mucilaginous, nervine, sedative. Root—anti-inflammatory, antispasmodic, anodyne, diuretic, nervine, pectoral, vulnerary. Cooling and moistening. Avoid while pregnant or breastfeeding. The seeds are poisonous.

Yerba Santa
(*Eriodictyon californicum*)

The name *yerba santa* means "holy herb," and it has a long history of use as an altar offering. Traditionally used as a reinforcer and cleanser of spirit, yerba santa is a natural repellant of stagnant and harmful energies. It is peaceful, nurturing, and capable of raising vibrations. Those who practice trance, meditation, and astral projection will find an encouraging ally in yerba santa. It is truly an amazing healer beneficial for shadow work and the releasing of trauma. Before beginning heavy emotional work, burn yerba santa and meditate on the courageous and revelatory magick of Kenaz.

Medicinal Properties
Yerba santa is a powerful expectorant and valued remedy for asthma. It's an antiseptic and diuretic and aids in the treatment of urinary complaints. The antiseptic qualities are also beneficial for sore throats and throat infections. The herb is useful for stimulating salivation, aiding in proper digestion, and alleviating muscle spasms. A poultice made from yerba santa is great for treating skin irritations like bruises, sprains, bug bites, and rashes. Actions: alterative, antiseptic, aromatic, carminative, decongestant, diuretic, expectorant. Warming and drying.

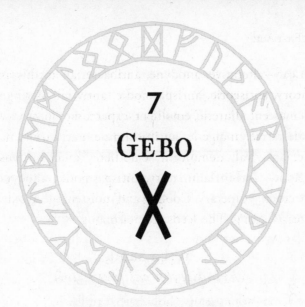

7
GEBO
ᚷ

Phonetic equivalent: Hard G
Gift, Equilibrium, Exchange

We must give if we take
For our well-being's sake
If we take, we must offer
In order to prosper

Gebo (pronounced Gee-boh) is the "gift" rune representing equilibrium, reciprocity, balance, exchange, and generosity. To the ancient Norse the act of gift giving was an important social convention. To be on the receiving end of a gift meant that one was also receiving an obligation for reciprocation. Not meeting this expectation was viewed as a sign of disrespect and could have serious consequences. It is believed that the willingness to be so giving came from the need to help each other during the harshness of winter, when food would have been most scarce.

Gebo relates to the Eastern concept of karma, which is a metaphysical principle of cause and effect. This principle states that the actions and intentions of an individual influence their future. A thoughtful adage regarding karma states that one tree can make one million matchsticks and one matchstick can burn down one million trees; meaning things tend to come around full circle sooner or later.

Magickally, Gebo is the giving and receiving of energies and ritualistic offerings for the entities with whom we work. Unlike the ancient social convention of gift giving, however, giving should not always come with expectation. Purely transactional relationships work best in the world of business. When it comes to relationships of love and respect, giving simply for the sake of it serves to deepen trust and bonds. When the ancient Norse peoples called on assistance from the gods they performed *blots,* or ritual blood sacrifices. During blots, it was common to sacrifice animals, but human lives were occasionally offered as well. Modern blots tend toward offerings of alcohol and food in place of ritual killing. While the type of offerings in blots have changed, what remains the same is the premise of balanced trade.

Because of its shape, Gebo cannot be drawn reversed or murkstave, but that is not to say the gift rune is immune from adversity. Revenge is considered an adverse action of Gebo, as well as theft and even the act of giving too much. Those who find it difficult to say *no* and allow themselves to be taken advantage of suffer from imbalanced Gebo. Derogatory terms for this type of personality are *doormat* or *pushover* and suggest a person's inability to disappoint others, even if it means causing stress or harm to themselves.

Rather than invoking the power of Gebo to better connect with nature, I view Gebo as more of an *outcome* of doing so—as a goal of rewilding. When we allow the pure wildness of Mother Earth to pervade our lives and become a regular part of it, we do ourselves a great service. For many, when it comes to technology versus nature, there is a steep imbalance in favor of technology. I do not view this as a fault but rather an inevitable outcome of the world in which we live. We all know that getting outside is good for our well-being, but just how good? According to a PBS article by Jim Robbins:

In a study of 20,000 people, a team led by Mathew White of the European Centre for Environment & Human Health at the University of Exeter found that people who spent two hours a week in green spaces—local parks or other natural environments, either all at once or spaced over several visits—were substantially more likely to report good health and psychological well-being than those who don't. Two hours was a hard boundary: The study showed there were no benefits for people who didn't meet that threshold.*

With the aid of Gebo, we can seek out and maintain balance between the spiritual world and the physical world so that we can, in turn, support the well-being of our whole selves. The following is an incense blend that, when burned, energetically takes on the essence of equilibrium and harmony:

∽ Gebo incense ∾

Gebo incense supports balance of mind, body, and spirit. Burn this blend when emotions are running high or when generally feeling out of sorts. It is a wonderful tool for meditation as it promotes calmness and clarity. Prepare during a first or third quarter moon, equinoxes are a perfect time as well, to increase the infusion of balanced energies. The following items are needed:

> Benzoin resin
> Dried forsythia flowers
> Dried lavender flowers (feel free to substitute or add any other herbs or resins that you find balancing in energy)
> Mortar and pestle
> Small piece of paper or dried leaf
> Pen or marker
> Empty jar

With a mortar and pestle, grind down the ingredients as best as you can. While doing so, focus on the overall intention of each ingredient as well as the finished product. Mix the ingredients well and pour half of the blend into an empty jar. With a writing utensil and a small piece of paper or dried leaf, draw the Gebo rune on both sides. You may choose to intone the name of the rune while doing so or to

---

*Jim Robbins, "How Immersing Yourself in Nature Benefits Your Health." *PBS News Hour* (website), January 13, 2020.

simply remain focused on the energies with which you wish to imbue the incense. Feel free to state an incantation like the following:

> *Powers of Gebo*
> *Balanced and fair*
> *Please bless this blend*
> *That I create with care*

Place the Gebo drawing in the jar on top of incense. Pour the remaining incense on top of the drawing. The paper or leaf should now be in the center of the blend. Close the jar and allow it to charge for an even number of days, preferably four. When ready for use, burn on a charcoal for best results. Hail, Gebo!

CORRESPONDENCES OF GEBO

ELEMENT	Air
ZODIAC	Libra
PLANET	Jupiter
MOON PHASE	First or Third Quarter
TAROT	Temperance, 6 of Cups
CRYSTAL	Banded Agate
CHAKRA	Heart
DEITIES	Baphomet, Kuan Yin, Ma'at, Ochosi, Odin
PLANTS	Ashwagandha, Benzoin, Forsythia, Ginseng, Lavender, Maple

The corresponding herbs of Gebo promote the increase of harmonious and balanced energies—something we all need for healing and general well-being. Gebo helps to foster the proper mindset needed to perform successful magick.

Ashwagandha
(*Withania somnifera*)

Ashwagandha is an adaptogen, which is a type of plant used medicinally to balance the body's systems. Such powers may be used magickally

to help one in attaining harmony within oneself and relationships—
especially relationships between humans and the divine. When our
thoughts and emotions become scattered, ashwagandha helps to ground
by promoting focus and calm. When feeling off kilter, add a pinch of
powdered ashwagandha to a carrier oil such as sunflower, olive, or coco-
nut, and trace Gebo over your third eye, heart, and solar plexus chakras.
I sometimes add a couple of pinches of the powdered root to my morning breakfast, tea, or smoothie.

Medicinal Properties

The root of ashwagandha, which is a staple in ayurvedic medicine, is
truly a magnificent remedy. It helps the mind, body, and spirit to adapt
to stress while promoting a balancing of bodily processes. Ashwagandha
is a rejuvenative capable of combating fatigue, inducing sleep, and boosting the immune system. It has long been used to treat male sexual issues
and increase sperm levels. As an anti-inflammatory, ashwagandha is an
excellent remedy for rheumatoid arthritis. It benefits fevers, ulcers, anemia, asthma, cancer, psoriasis, and tuberculosis. Actions: adaptogen,
alterative, analgesic, antidepressant, anti-inflammatory, antispasmodic,
aphrodisiac, nervine, nootropic, mild sedative, tonic. Warming. Use
with caution during pregnancy.

Benzoin
(*Styrax benzoin*)

Benzoin is a resin gathered from *Styrax* trees such as Japanese snow-
bell. It attracts success, blesses spaces (like new homes, for example),
purifies, and banishes. It promotes improved mood and aids those on
the path of spiritual alchemy. When we embark on astral journeys, it
is paramount that we prepare ourselves to expect the unexpected and
be ready for anything, as we do not know what is waiting for us as we
navigate different realms. The earthy resin strengthens the mind while
also shielding the traveler from ill-intentioned energies and spirits. It
is of the utmost importance, when doing magick of this sort, that one
is balanced in mind, body, and spirit, and benzoin can help one attain
such stability. Going into the unknown while angry, sad, fatigued, or ill

creates disadvantage and leaves one vulnerable in uncharted territory. Burn benzoin and add Gebo to a bindrune with Raidho, Kenaz, and Elhaz when preparing to journey to other realms.

Medicinal Properties

Benzoin is a natural antibiotic commonly applied as a topical remedy for a variety of skin conditions such as sores, cuts, and blisters. Add to vaporizers to soothe laryngitis, sore throats, and lung congestion. Benzoin may be taken internally as an antiseptic for urinary infections but should only be done so under the supervision of a healthcare professional. Benzoin supports oral hygiene and is often added to mouthwash to tighten gums and kill the bacteria that causes bad breath. The astringent properties that tighten the gums are also beneficial for toning the skin. The essential oil helps to alleviate pain and stiffness of the joints and muscles. In aromatherapy the oil is used to treat anxiety and mild depression. Actions: anti-inflammatory, antiseptic, astringent, expectorant, mild stimulant. Warming and moistening.

Forsythia
(*Forsythia* spp.)

Forsythia flowers have four petals—four being symbolic of stability, balance, and a strong foundation. The number four and nature go hand in hand, made evident by the elements, cardinal directions, seasons, and phases of the moon. Burn in incense blends when feeling imbalanced in body, mind, or spirit. When given as a gift, forsythia grants the recipient with vibrant solar energy, supporting confidence, optimism, good health, and success.

Medicinal Properties

Common ailments for which forsythia is used include fever, skin irritations, parasites, muscle pain, and bacterial infections. The fruit, known as Lian Qiao in traditional Chinese medicine, is valued for its anti-inflammatory properties, which target excess heat and swelling. They have also been used to assist in the removal of bodily toxins, for the treatment of respiratory complaints, and to ease nausea. Actions: anti-bacterial, anti-inflammatory, antioxidant, antiviral, diuretic, emmenagogue, febrifuge, vermifuge, vulnerary. Cooling. Forsythia may slow the clotting of blood and should be avoided before surgery and by those on anti-coagulant medications. Avoid during pregnancy and nursing.

Ginseng
(*Panax ginseng*)

Ginseng is a true panacea. In China, conflicts have arisen in an effort to gain control of the forests in which it is found. Because its extensive list of health benefits is often highlighted, ginseng is rarely found in *materia magickas,* but it is indeed a powerful plant in many ways. *The Herbal Alchemist's Handbook* by Karen Harrison points out its benefits for sex and love, stating that one can inscribe the name of their intended partner on one side of the root and their name on the other, followed by enveloping it in red cloth and visualizing the desired union.* While ginseng would make sense paired with a more amorous rune, I've chosen to include it with Gebo due to its all-around affinity for balance, that is, balanced health, balanced love, balanced *life.* Ginseng is a big picture plant. In magick, we can take advantage of its ability as a balancer and apply that power to a number of spells, rituals, formulas, and charms. It's magickal and medical uses are one and the same and should be employed to bring harmony where it is needed.

Medicinal Properties

This remarkable plant has been prized for thousands of years for strengthening in cases of debility, illness, or weakness due to old age. It works to improve stamina, immunity, liver function, memory, and cognitive function while helping the body adapt to a variety of stressors in order to regain homeostasis. Ginseng eases the symptoms of menopause. It has a long history of being used to remedy erectile dysfunction. This amazing plant is believed to have strong anticancer properties, but more research is needed. Actions: adaptogen, anti-inflammatory, antioxidant, demulcent, hypertensive, immunostimulant, nootropic, stimulant, rejuvenative, tonic. Warming and moistening.

---

*Karen Harrison, *The Herbal Alchemist's Handbook: A Complete Guide to Magickal Herbs and How to Use Them* (Newburyport, Mass.: Weiser Books, 2020), 152.

Lavender
(*Lavandula angustifolia, officinalis*)

Lavender is one of the most adored herbs available today. Because of its unique scent and relaxing properties, it is frequently added to skin-care, candles, fragrances, teas, and even stuffed animals! It covers a wide range of possible uses such as love, tranquillity, healing, protection, purification, and visionary work. Lavender offers stability, peace, and clarity of mind. Bathe in the flower buds or place some inside your pillowcase for a deeply peaceful sleep. Keep lavender around the home to promote a happy household and fidelity among lovers. While its energies are calm and soft, lavender is genuinely strengthening and especially protective of those suffering from abuse. I have included lavender in Gebo's garden due to its varying abilities—like adaptogens, lavender is well rounded and works to keep the spirit, mind, and body balanced. Its power is often called on to assist with spiritual growth and healing. Interestingly, *Magical Herbalism* by Scott Cunningham recommends carrying the herb to see ghosts!

Medicinal Properties

As a nervine and mild analgesic, lavender is a wonderful additive in tea and tincture blends for headaches, especially headaches brought on by stress. Combine with feverfew and take regularly to prevent cluster headaches. The diluted essential oil may be applied to the forehead, temples, and back of neck to relieve tension. In any form it relaxes the high-strung, type A personality and benefits those with anxiety and depression. The essential oil soothes hives, burns, and cracked skin. Bathe infants in lavender to soothe colic and promote restful sleep. Actions: analgesic, antibacterial, antifungal, anti-inflammatory, aromatic, bronchodilator, carminative, cholagogue, diuretic, nervine, rejuvenative. Cooling and drying.

Maple
(*Acer* spp.)

As a tree of balanced feminine and masculine energies, healing, longevity, and protection, it's no wonder the wood is so popular in the making of wands. It aids in the rebalancing of a person, place, or object after the removal of evil spirits. In general, trees are symbols of wisdom and protection, and maple is no exception; add bits of bark to incense and burn while meditating on the big questions regarding life, death, and spirit. If you have access to a maple tree, a Gebo stave can be created with two fallen twigs and a bit of twine. Because of its natural sweetness, maple syrup makes a wonderful offering to deities and ancestors alike.

Medicinal Properties

The syrup of the sugar maple is a delicious remedy for cough and sore throat. The leaves and inner bark support spleen, gallbladder, and liver health. A poultice made from the bark and leaves may be applied externally to relieve wounds, joint pain, and swelling. In Western Europe during the Middle Ages maple leaves were added to hot baths or kept on the soles of the feet to relieve stubborn fevers. Actions: analgesic, anti-inflammatory, antiseptic, diuretic, febrifuge, hepatoprotective, sedative.

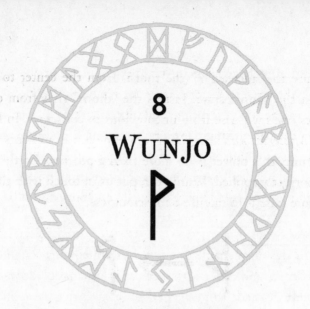

8
WUNJO

ᚹ

Phonetic equivalent: W, V
Joy, Will, Perfection

Smile upon me Wunjo
Bless me with a joyful soul
Shine on me from Valhalla
With glistening rays of gold

Wunjo (pronounced woon-yo) is the eighth and final rune of Freyja's aett. It embodies genuine joy and wish fulfillment. While some runes are quite complex in their meanings, I find Wunjo to be quite simple and straightforward. With happiness and wish fulfillment at its helm, it has undeniable associations with Christmas, particularly Santa Claus—a mythical character possibly based in part on Odin, the bearded Norse god who flies through the night sky on his eight-legged horse, Sleipnir, delivering gifts or punishments to children. Those who support the theory of Santa's evolution from Odin suggest that the eight legs of Sleipnir over time transformed into the eight flying reindeer we are familiar with today.

Wunjo is happiness, innocence, compassion, peace, and perfection. Its shape and correlation to the Thurisaz rune illustrates the raising of vibrations. You may recall, one of the meanings of Thurisaz is the shadow or unconscious will. Imagine the Thurisaz stave in your mind's eye and raise the sideways *V* (the thorn) from the center to the top, resulting in the Wunjo stave. Just as the "thorn" rises from center to top, so does one's will rise from unconscious to conscious. In her book *Northern Mysteries and Magick,* Freya Aswynn comments, "In the Thurisaz rune, this power is no more than a potential in the subconscious. If correctly applied, Wunjo can put us in touch with this power and therefore raise it to manifest consciousness."*

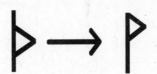

In a reading, the appearance of Wunjo is reassurance that one is on the right path—making healthy decisions and prioritizing the well-being of the self and others. The surrounding runes may indicate that which does, or can, create real happiness in one's life. When pulled alongside runes such as Nauthiz or Hagalaz, Wunjo may bring the message that *this, too, shall pass.* A pairing of Wunjo and Perthro may be a reminder to not take life too seriously. Reversed or murkstave the joy rune can point to misery, loneliness, loss of interest, or disconnection to one's true will or higher values. If reversed Wunjo comes up in a reading, it's probably best to hold off on the making of important decisions.

Wunjo represents the power of seeing the glass as half full and the ability to find the silver linings within difficulties. It is healthy positivity and never toxic positivity. Call on the rune of joy when seeking out your highest will or when a more optimistic view would be beneficial.

Through Wunjo we can better connect to nature through the art of "not taking things too seriously." For some, this is a concept that must be practiced. When I think of not taking life too seriously, I recall something a dear friend told me about a camping trip she went on with three other companions. Once the group reached their campsite, they

---

*Freya Aswynn, *Northern Mysteries and Magick: Runes & Feminine Powers* (Woodbury, Minn.: Llewellyn Publications, 2003), 38.

split into pairs to erect two tents. Both pairs were having tremendous trouble doing so, but each handled the difficulties very differently; one pair got increasingly frustrated and angry while my friend and her partner found themselves laughing and joking at their mishaps. This simple story has stuck with me after many years. It highlighted to me the importance of seeing through the lens of humor and lightheartedness. Why sweat the small things? Intellectually we understand the importance, but sometimes life operates in a manner just annoying enough to make us forget and want to set a tent on fire.

As someone who has long "taken things too seriously," I make a point of trying to never forget the importance of the phrase "fuck it" paired with a good laugh. In terms of magick, we learn early on about the law of attraction and how like attracts like. If we are miserable, we will inevitably continue to view the world as a miserable place full of sorrow. If we are optimistic and empathetic, we will easily see the good in others and attract auspicious energies. This is not to say, of course, that undesirable situations will never again befall one who maintains a sense of optimism, but rather, someone who maintains a positive mental attitude is more likely to find solutions and silver linings within their difficulties. The narratives we make up between our ears have the power to shape our lives.

Many years ago, a different friend of mine woke up in the morning to see that his car had been stolen in the night. *I* was positively furious for him. He filed a police report, but to my surprise, seemed largely unaffected. "Why aren't you pissed?" I demanded of him. He looked at me, shrugged his shoulders, and said, "Because in a year from now, this isn't going to matter." Insert image of me with my jaw hitting the floor.

My friend's incredibly wise answer made a huge impression on me, and when something goes wrong in my life, I stop and ask myself, "Will this matter to me one year from now?" Often, the answer is no, and it saves me a lot of grief. Stress and anger have a tremendous impact on the mind, body, and spirit. We can become physically ill, fatigued, depressed, anxious . . . or we could choose to react to common stressors like my friend, who never lost a wink of sleep over that car, which was never found, by the way. If the answer to "will this matter to me one year from now?" is yes, then that's a different story. It helps no one to try to put a positive spin on a tragedy or deep injustice, and that is not the message I wish to put out here. Grief and anger have their places.

So how can all this help us better connect to nature? When we do our best to maintain encouraging outlooks, we in turn take better care of ourselves; we place importance on a sense of overall well-being. Someone who prioritizes self-care is more likely to get outside and enjoy the simple things.

Learning to get a handle on our emotions is so vital to a healthy existence; otherwise we are knocked around life like a pinball, always bouncing from one unpleasant situation and emotion to the next. Low vibrations attract low vibrations. So next time you find yourself in a particularly annoying situation, call on the power of Wunjo for wisdom and guidance; and don't forget to ask yourself, "Will this matter one year from now?" Hail, Wunjo!

CORRESPONDENCES OF WUNJO

ELEMENT	Air
ZODIAC	Leo
PLANET	Sun, Jupiter
MOON PHASE	Waxing, Full
TAROT	The Star
CRYSTAL	Bornite
CHAKRA	Heart
DEITIES	Cocamama, Hathor, Lalita, Uzume
PLANTS	Anise, Carnation, Lemon Balm, Marshmallow, Meadowsweet, Olive, Sunflower

The corresponding plants of Wunjo are strong advocates of PMA (Positive Mental Attitude). Apply to magickal workings that seek to reduce and heal anxiety, sadness, and depression.

Anise
(*Pimpinella anisum*)

True anise, not to be confused with star anise, is commonly used as a flavoring agent. It reminds me of my nana, who often baked with it and made the world's best terrelles (my nana's spelling of tarralis) and pizzelles. The smell alone takes me back to my grandparents' house on Christmas Eve. Aside from Italian baked goods, its uplifting flavor is commonly added to wedding and handfasting cakes. Its natural sweetness is perfect for teas, tinctures, elixirs, and other herbal remedies. Anise isn't only for those about to tie the knot; it also plays Cupid for those hoping to welcome romance into their lives. To encourage sweet dreams, sprinkle anise seeds inside of your pillowcase just before bedtime. Powdered, it may be added to incense for the honoring of one's beloved dead. Additional talents include warding against the evil eye and activation of psychic ability. Add to a ritual bath before divinatory practices.

Medicinal Properties

Anise is an excellent source of antioxidants, which help prevent cellular damage and premature aging of the skin. Its antifungal properties are effective against yeast infections. The seeds are used to relieve gas and digestive upset and are gentle enough for infants with colic. When taken as a hot tea, it helps to soothe coughs and relieve chest congestion. Anise stimulates menstruation and the production of breast milk. Its wide range of remedial uses covers mild urinary tract infections, dysmenorrhea, asthma, lice, and scabies. Use topically to soothe the pain of arthritis. Actions: antibacterial, antifungal, antispasmodic, antiviral, aromatic, carminative, digestive, diuretic, emmenagogue, estrogenic, expectorant, pectoral, stimulant, vermifuge. Warming. Avoid during pregnancy.

Carnation
(*Dianthus caryophyllus*)

Carnation's Latin binomial literally translates to "Flower of God," a name bestowed upon it by the Greek philosopher Theophrastus.

Because carnations are available in so many colors, they offer a variety of uses: pink represents familial and friend love, white is associated with peace and purity, and purple represents prosperity and honor. Regardless of color, carnations help to raise the vibrations and instill hope. Adding flowers to a bath encourages an enhanced mood. Carnation promotes joy and laughter and is wonderful for the mending of strained relationships.

Medicinal Properties

While medicinal usage of carnation is now obsolete, it was once applied to a range of afflictions. Traditionally the flowers were used to treat fevers, cough, and colds and were ingested as a tonic for liver and heart health. In traditional Chinese medicine, carnation was used to expel parasites. The essential oil benefits various skin conditions, relieves sore muscles, and soothes anxiety and mild depression. Actions: alexiteric, anti-inflammatory, antispasmodic, aromatic, diaphoretic, nervine, stimulant, vermifuge.

Lemon Balm
(*Melissa officinalis*)

Lemon balm has a special place in my heart. Not only is it one of the first plants I learned about when I began my herbal studies, it's also the first plant I really sat and meditated with. What I learned from my early meditations with lemon balm is how uplifting and gentle it really is. *Melissa* from its Latin name translates to "bee." Bees were said to be messengers of goddesses; therefore, lemon balm is known for imparting wisdom and love. It strengthens the bonds of any relationship including romances, friendships, and familial love. It's a go-to herb for workings of healing, romance, and sensuality. In medieval times, it was used to drive away evil spirits. As an herb of the moon, lemon balm is sacred to the Roman lunar goddess Diana. Bathe in its leaves to promote self-love and confidence and to banish melancholy. Its ability to calm the body and mind makes this uplifting herb a true ally for those who practice meditation and trance work.

Medicinal Properties

The alchemist Paracelsus spoke highly of lemon balm, calling it an "elixir of life." He believed it had the power of revitalization and longevity. Gentle and calming, it promotes relaxation for those who suffer from anxiety, hyperactivity, nervous stomach, and insomnia. It is especially helpful for children who are unable to calm down at bedtime. Lemon balm balances thyroid function, strengthens memory, relieves headaches and migraines, detoxifies the liver, and reduces symptoms of PMS. As an antiviral, it is an effective treatment for cold sores. Actions: antibacterial, anticancer, antidepressant, antihistamine, anti-inflammatory, antioxidant, antispasmodic, antiviral, aromatic, carminative, cholagogue, diaphoretic, digestive, emmenagogue, febrifuge, hepatoprotective, nervine, nootropic, sedative, vasodilator. Cooling. Avoid alongside thyroid medications.

Marshmallow
(*Althaea officinalis*)

The lovely perennial that is marshmallow is a plant of friendship and works quite well to repair strained or injured relationships. As a natural lubricant, its energies work to smooth things over. Gifted to a friend, the flower is a symbol of forgiveness and reconciliation. Marshmallow, like marjoram, is a plant of love and death, often used to honor deceased loved ones and attract kindly spirits.

Medicinal Properties

Marshmallow root's primary healing powers come from its cooling and mucilaginous properties. Drinking a cold infusion of the root eases sore throat and dry cough. Boiling the roots in milk and honey helps to effectively treat bronchitis. Marshmallow relieves congestion of the sinuses and lungs. It is soothing for skin conditions such as sunburn, bug bites, burns, hives, eczema, psoriasis, and dandruff. As a galactagogue, marshmallow enriches breastmilk production. Actions: alterative, anti-inflammatory, demulcent, diuretic, emollient, expectorant, galactagogue, nutritive, pulmonary, vulnerary. Cooling and moistening. Avoid while pregnant or before surgery. If diabetic, check with a health-care professional before use.

Meadowsweet
(*Filipendula ulmaria*)

It is said that where meadowsweet grows, wickedness cannot thrive. It radiates peace and joy and effortlessly protects against harmful entities. Meadowsweet, which was sacred to the ancient Druids, is an herb of compassion and love and works well for spells regarding romance, friendship, and family. Traditionally, it has been used as a strewing herb due to its alluring floral aroma. Burn the dried herb as incense to energetically cleanse a space after a heated argument. Drink an infusion to raise personal vibrations and cleanse the spirit body. Infusions are also ideal for bathing crystals, altars, or anything (or anyone) that seems to have inadvertently picked up unfavorable energies.

Medicinal Properties
Meadowsweet is an antacid that helps relieve heartburn and acid reflux. It supports healthy digestion and remedies diarrhea. Meadowsweet contains salicylic acid, which treats colds and fevers and served as the forerunner to aspirin. It effectively targets arthritis and minor pains. In the UK, it was added to rainwater, which was then used as a toner for the skin. Actions: analgesic, antacid, antibacterial, anti-inflammatory, aromatic, astringent, diaphoretic, diuretic, stomachic. Cooling and drying. Large doses may cause vomiting.

Olive
(*Olea europaea*)

The olive tree is a totem of Greece, and the branch is a universal symbol of peace. The well-known phrase "to extend an olive branch" refers to the reconciliation between two parties who were once at odds with one another. Olive is sacred to the goddess Athena and is a symbol of divine wisdom and blessings. Its sunny energies are happy, harmonious, and hopeful. The widely used cooking oil may be used to draw magickal symbols on the body during ritual. It is also a popular base for ritual oils and adds its own brand of sun-ruled protection to blends. Olives are perfect offerings for deities of Egyptian, Greek, and Roman pantheons.

Medicinal Properties

Olives are rich in antioxidants, vitamin E, and heart-healthy fats. The leaves of the olive tree may be used to lower blood pressure and improve circulatory function. They also treat angina and lower blood sugar. The leaves are mildly antiviral and antibacterial. Combine and ingest olive oil and lemon juice followed by plenty of water to help break down and clear kidney stones. Olive oil is mildly laxative. Actions: antioxidant, antiviral, diuretic, febrifuge, hypotensive, nutritive. Cooling and drying. The leaves are astringent and antiseptic. The oil is demulcent and laxative.

Sunflower
(*Helianthus annuus*)

The radiant, towering sunflower invokes all the bright energies of the sun: health, vitality, happiness, success, confidence, and higher will. At first, I placed this flower with Sowilo the sun rune, but I find that it works just as well with Wunjo. After all, Wunjo's planetary correspondence is the sun. Ritual baths filled with sunflower combat depression and low self-esteem while promoting inner strength and zest for life. It is fitting for workings on Sundays, sabbat celebrations, and of course for working alongside solar deities. Sunflowers encourage individuality and a balanced solar plexus chakra. In some magickal traditions women were encouraged to eat the seeds during the waxing moon to help them become pregnant. Like olive, sunflower's oil is an excellent carrier for essential oil blends.

Medicinal Properties

Sunflowers are rich in vitamins A, D, and E and are excellent additions to skin moisturizers. The oil soothes eczema, psoriasis, and lesions, and relieves constipation when taken internally. A poultice of the leaves is best for snake or spider bites. Tea made from the leaves helps to relieve fevers. The seeds are high in dietary fiber and are helpful in reducing stress and anxiety. Actions: Leaves—anti-inflammatory, astringent, diuretic, expectorant, febrifuge. Drying. Actions: Seeds—diuretic, expectorant, immunostimulant.

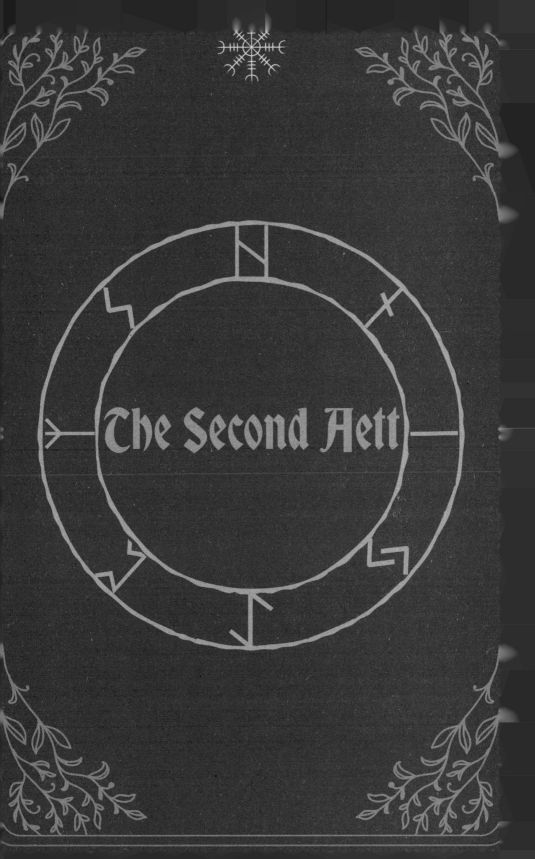

The Second Aett

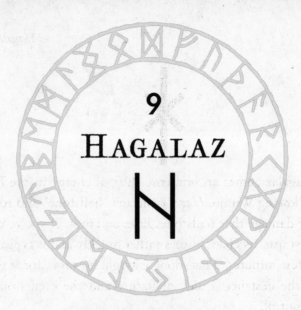

9
HAGALAZ

Phonetic equivalent: H
Hail, Chaos, Destruction

Stones of ice that rain destruction
A volcano's violent eruption
Great Hagalaz and stormy power
I invoke thee at this witching hour

Hagalaz (pronounced hah-gah-lahz), which translates to "hail," is the ninth rune of the Elder Futhark and marks the beginning of the second aett, called Hagall's aett—Hagall being an alternative name for Hagalaz. Its position at number nine indicates Hagalaz's importance among the runes. In Norse mythology, nine is a holy number and appears in much of the lore. When Odin hung from the World Tree (which contains nine worlds) he did so for nine days and nights. During Ragnarök, in his final battle, Thor takes nine steps before he is defeated by the serpent Jörmungandr. These are just a few examples of the many nines throughout the mythology.

The order of the runes is not arbitrary. There is good reason why Hagalaz holds the ninth, or sacred, position. In its alternative form (see figure p. 101) Hagalaz is known as the seed that contains within it the energies of all the runes. It is the catalyst for gaining strength, wisdom, and growth.

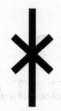

With Hagalaz comes an immense shift of energy in the Futhark, especially following Wunjo. *Hagalaz* means "hailstone" and represents the threat of damage that hailstones have on crops. If you've ever witnessed a hailstorm, its chaos ensues rather quickly and is typically over after only a few minutes. That's long enough, however, for it to wreak havoc. It is the destructive side of nature and the events outside of humanity's control.

While writing this section, I experienced the worst hailstorm I'd seen in many years. Where I live in the northeastern United States, hailstorms are a very rare occurrence, so it felt like a good omen to experience Hagalaz in action as I write this; although, the plants in my garden probably don't share the same sentiments.

When nature rears up in such a way, it's truly fascinating and frightening at the same time. When we experience floods, earthquakes, tornadoes, and the like, we simply have to wait them out and hope for the best. Just as Mother Nature experiences Hagalaz, so do we on personal levels. Spiritual awakening often follows major crisis and radical change; destruction and transformation that inevitably lead to rebirth. It is the beginning of the alchemical process; the *solve* before the *coagula*. Hail, which can be harmful to plant life, eventually melts and becomes nourishment for the same beings it once threatened to destroy.

Hagalaz is the rune of Hel, the half-dead daughter of the god Loki as well as the name of the underworld she rules over. Hel is not to be confused with the Christian hell, which is a place of suffering and punishment; rather Hel is a neutral underworld for the dead who did not die in battle. Those who did die in battle, of course, go to Odin's Valhalla or Freyja's Fólkvangr.

This rune and the next two are associated with the Norns—three giantess women who live at the base of the Yggdrasil (World Tree) and control every living being's past, present, and future via the web of

Wyrd. Urd, the eldest Norn and ruler of the past, is specific to Hagalaz. In terms of witchcraft, Hagalaz is the dark aspect of feminine magick and is valuable for shadow work, protection, hexing, cursing, and rising from particularly low points in one's life. It is a reminder that enduring hardship is a necessary step for achieving change and the strength to move on. In readings, there are no reversed or murkstave meanings.

When I first began working with the runes, I was a bit intimidated by Hagalaz. If it appeared in a reading, I became uneasy. Now, however, I have learned to embrace Hagalaz. It is not a "bad" rune, just as hail isn't "bad"—it's just a natural process. Like everything in nature, we cannot file the runes under such oversimplified classifications. They all have their place and importance. Without the difficulties of Hagalaz we can never truly appreciate the blessings of Wunjo.

I have come to know Hagalaz as a symbol of empowerment. When I think back over the seemingly terrible things that have happened in my life, I'm able to find reason, and even appreciation, in hindsight. We are all undoubtedly stronger and wiser because of our troubles. For many years I struggled with alcohol addiction and severe depression. In the final years of active addiction, I found myself drowning in utter hopelessness desperately grasping for a life raft. After many failed attempts of getting sober, I found relief in Buddhism, which inevitably brought me back to witchcraft. Buddhism and witchcraft were among the things that saved my life. Years later I find myself sober, healthy, confident, and hopeful for the future. I mean, I'm sitting here writing a book. Amazing! I no longer regret my struggles because they have led me to (or rather, mercilessly dragged me to) a higher path. *This* is Hagalaz! It is scary, fortifying, and revelatory. It is the impetus to great progress.

Hagalaz teaches us to connect to nature with pure authenticity. It demands that we seek out, confront, and release the weights that hold us down and keep us from moving forward. Do keep in mind, however, that confronting the memories and beliefs that continue to cause suffering is a heavy task, and for some it is best done with the help of a mentor, counselor, or therapist.

To heal the mind and spirit, it is best to start small rather than to dive right into the deep psychological traumas. Affirmations, which are nothing more than encouraging declarations, are an effective way to dip your toes into the vast waters of healing and self-love. Statements as simple as "I forgive myself," "I am worthy of love," or "I am resilient" can go a long way. Look in the mirror when you tell yourself these things and don't forget to *mean* them.

Hagalaz is raw, real, and tough as nails, and it supports us in finding personal sovereignty through authenticity. This rune has no patience for dishonesty or self-deprecation. When we dishonor the self, we dishonor the spirit of Hagalaz, which teaches us to accept ourselves for exactly who we are, flaws and all! We are manifestations of cosmic energy in search of alignment and purpose. As long as we are seeking we are succeeding. We are never visitors of nature; we *are* nature. When we peel back all the layers of what it means to be human, at the very core we are children of Earth and Spirit. Love yourself like your life depends on it!

The following is a simple ritual meant to release what holds us back. It is best performed at night during a full or waning moon, preferably in a secluded outside area.

What you'll need:

A dried leaf or sheet of bark. I personally prefer dried bay leaves. If these aren't available to you, paper works fine.
A marker or pen
Matches or a lighter
About a cup of water. Rain, moon, or snow water are best and if possible, melted hail water is even better!
A cauldron, bowl, or small saucepan
An outdoor spot where you can dig a small hole in the soil

On the dried leaf or paper, write down a word or small phrase that represents that which you wish to remove from your life. What is holding you back from reaching your full potential? What is keeping you from accepting yourself wholly? Are there any cycles of pain that tend to be repeated in your life? Work from these questions. If you're not sure, it may be helpful to do a bit of introspective journaling first.

To begin, position the cauldron or bowl in front of you and recite the following:

Alchemy of Hagalaz
Let this hindrance burn
Let the smoke whisk it away
Allow it never to return

Hold the leaf (or paper) on which you've written directly above the cauldron or bowl and very carefully ignite it. Once the fire catches, drop it into the vessel. Move your attention to the smoke and visualize that which you've banished being carried far away with the smoke. Once the burning is complete, pour the water into the vessel and onto your hands. You are symbolically cleansing yourself of that which you've released. Dig a small hole in the soil, pour in the water and ashes from your vessel, and recover the soil. Seal the ritual with a closing statement such as "it is done," "and so it is," "so mote it be," or "Hail, Hagalaz!"

CORRESPONDENCES OF HAGALAZ

ELEMENT	Ice
ZODIAC	Scorpio
PLANET	Saturn
MOON PHASE	Dark
TAROT	The Tower, The Devil
CRYSTAL	Hematite
CHAKRA	Root
DEITIES	Baba Yaga, Hekate, Kali, Lilith, Nicneven, Oya
PLANTS	Asafoetida, Blackthorn, Centaury, Deadly Nightshade, Foxglove, Hellebore, Wormwood

The corresponding herbs of Hagalaz are valuable for those who wish to engage in self-acceptance, shadow work, or to celebrate their authenticity. They are formidable herbs, capable of empowering, protecting, or harming.

Asafoetida
(*Ferula asafoetida*)

Asafoetida is an acrid resin that is often powdered and burned in rituals of cleansing and banishing, especially in cases of evil spirits. Its scent is, in my opinion, quite foul and does a good job of banishing *me* out of any room in which it burns. (I personally recommend burning it outside!) Its charming moniker, devil's dung, is no doubt a result of its sulfurous odor. Asafoetida's potent exorcising power aids one in discarding their own harmful habits and desires. One of its traditional uses includes keeping it on one's person to repel the evil eye and law enforcement. The powder is an essential safety measure to keep nearby for any practitioners who dabble in spirit conjuring and necromancy.

Medicinal Properties

Asafoetida supports gastrointestinal health and works wonders for bloating, gas, and indigestion. It helps to clear out congested lungs as well as intestinal tracts. Today, asafoetida is mostly taken in supplement form for various respiratory troubles such as asthma, whooping cough, or bronchitis. Actions: antibacterial, anticancer, antioxidant, antispasmodic, carminative, digestive tonic, expectorant, laxative, sedative. Hot and drying. May be unsafe for children.

Blackthorn
(*Prunus spinosa*)

Similar to elder trees, blackthorn trees are known for establishing contact between humans and other realms, namely the faery realm. Its energies border mischievous and menacing, making it a frontrunner of plants in baneful magick. The subduing of one's enemies falls under the umbrella of blackthorns offenses. Conversely, it has also been used to ward off harmful energies and evil. Under the rulership of Saturn, this deciduous tree is ideal for creating boundaries symbolized by its common use as dividing hedge on property lines. It also aids the practitioner in shifting perspective and coming into their own power. It relates to protective and chthonic deities, clairvoyance, and the Celtic sabbat of Samhain. Blackthorn's sharp, spiny branches may be used to create a

Hagalaz stave, which can be hung outside the home to warn malicious people and spirits away.

Medicinal Properties

The berry of blackthorn (called sloe—as in sloe gin) and the dried flower have been used to remedy the common cold, cough, fatigue, constipation, inflammation of the mouth and throat, and more. It is a mild sedative with blood-cleansing properties. The bark and roots especially are highly astringent. Blackthorn berries are most commonly employed as a flavoring in herbal teas, syrups, wines, and liqueurs, specifically sloe gin. Actions: alterative, astringent, anti-inflammatory, diaphoretic, mild diuretic, laxative, mild sedative. Warming and drying. Use at your own risk. The safety of the blackthorn as a medicine has been questioned. The seeds contain cyanide. Unfortunately, there has not been a lot of study to confirm or refute any suspicions.

Centaury
(*Erythraea centaurium*)

The legendary Greek centaur Chiron, who makes up the constellation of Sagittarius, used this herb to heal a wound caused by a poisoned arrow. Similarly, today centaury is employed to rid a person or place of toxic energies, including anger, hostile magick, evil spirits, and the like. Like Chiron, as well as Hagalaz, centaury enjoys a reputation of great power, and can be added to any working to increase the effectiveness of the magick.

Medicinal Properties

Centaury is a wonderful bitter that may be taken before a meal to kickstart digestion. It is used for treating dyspepsia, stimulating appetite, and assimilating nutrients. It is cleansing to the blood, kidneys, and liver. Historically, it was used to treat jaundice, gout, and scurvy. For best results, centaury should be taken over the course of weeks. Actions: alterative, aromatic, bitter, digestive tonic, febrifuge, stomachic. Cooling.

Deadly Nightshade
(*Atropa belladonna*)

Deadly nightshade, or belladonna as it's also commonly known, is Hagalaz in plant form. She's beautiful, dangerous, and brimming with chthonic magick. She is of the underworld and may be used to curse an unfaithful partner or even attract a new one. Consuming the plant and its berries can cause hallucinations, severe headaches, seizures, and even death. Simply touching deadly nightshade can cause adverse skin affects; so if you choose to engage in her magick, please use caution and wear gloves! According to Norse lore, eating the berries, known in northern Europe as Walkerbeeren or *Valkyrie berry,* would bring death by the Valkyries themselves. Deadly nightshade is known as a main ingredient in Witches' Flying Ointment, which induced altered states and allowed witches to "fly" via its psychotropic properties. Its Latin name derives from the eldest Greek fate Atropos who, like the Norn Skuld, is the bringer of death.

Medicinal Properties
Due to its toxicity, deadly nightshade is not recommended for medicinal applications. Traditionally it was used for respiratory ailments and as a topical pain reliever. Actions: hallucinogenic, narcotic, soporific. Cooling and moistening. Highly toxic. For dosage information consult with a professional herbalist. Do not handle while pregnant or nursing.

Foxglove
(*Digitalis purpurea*)

Foxglove is a plant of the underworld and acts as a bridge for those brave enough to journey beyond the veil. It is an ally of the hedge witch who keeps one foot firmly planted in unearthly realms at all times. The energies of foxglove are protective, courageous, chthonic, and passionate. This treacherous beauty can act as a portal to the faery realm, and offerings to the fae are commonly placed within the bell-shaped flowers. Foxglove is said to be able to "raise the dead and kill the living."

Medicinal Properties

Due to its toxicity, foxglove is not recommended for medicinal usage. Historically it was used to treat congestive heart failure. Even small doses, however, can result in cardiac arrest.

Hellebore
(*Helleborus niger*)

In Greek, the word *helleborus* translates to "injure food," and even though this ominous plant can cause harm, it also has a history of use as a healer. In particular, the flower energetically aids in the soothing of mental turmoil. Keeping a hellebore amulet on oneself helps one to go unnoticed by others, which is particularly helpful for empaths or folks who suffer from social anxiety. It is associated with necromancy, chthonic goddesses, protection, exorcism, banishing, and the conjuring of demons. It can initiate or break curses. Like deadly nightshade, this member of the buttercup family was a staple in Witches' Flying Ointment. As a perennial that is both frost resistant and drought tolerant, hellebore symbolizes resilience.

Medicinal Properties

Due to its toxicity, hellebore is not recommended for medicinal usage. Traditionally it has been used to detoxify the body, reduce fevers, alleviate spasms, and treat dysmenorrhea. Actions: anti-inflammatory, antioxidant, sedative, vermifuge. Cooling and drying. For dosage information consult with a professional herbalist. Do not handle while pregnant or nursing.

Wormwood
(*Artemisia absinthium*)

Wormwood and its feminine counterpart mugwort were among the very first herbs to catch my attention when I began my studies in magickal herbalism. Their names alone conjure visions of bubbling cauldrons and antique cabinets overflowing with herbs, potions, and elixirs. Turns out I wasn't too far off, as the artemisias are incredibly potent and mystical herbs, steeped in enchantment and lore. Wormwood, which is the traditional main ingredient in absinthe, aids in clairvoyance, divination, necromancy, spells of vengeance, and astral travel. It is perfect for cleansing, banishing, exorcism, and relieving anger. Traditionally, this herb was thrown into Samhain bonfires to increase one's ability to see ghosts while providing protection from evil spirits. The synergy of Hagalaz and wormwood yields formidable energy, especially when worked during liminal periods that include the dark moon, full moon, eclipses, Beltane, or Samhain. According to legend, wormwood grew from the path of the serpent as it was cast out of the garden of Eden and is therefore sacred to the rebel goddess Lilith.

Medicinal Properties

Wormwood is mildly psychoactive due to the volatile oil thujone, which is also present in its close relative, mugwort. With the proper dose, this antiparasitic herb can be taken for colitis and nervous disorders, and to stimulate healthy appetite and digestion. Wormwood has long been utilized to relieve high fevers and eliminate intestinal parasites. In eastern Europe, it was traditionally used as a remedy for malaria. Actions: abortifacient, alterative, mild antidepressant, anti-inflammatory, antimicrobial, antiparasitic, aromatic, astringent, bitter, cholagogue, emmenagogue, febrifuge, stomachic, vermifuge. Cooling and drying. Wormwood should be used sparingly as it can have adverse effects. Cold. Avoid while pregnant or breastfeeding.

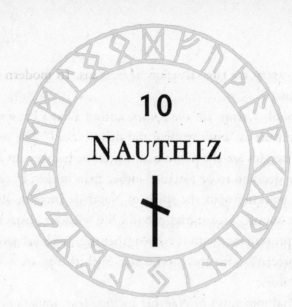

10
NAUTHIZ

Phonetic equivalent: N
Need, Sacrifice, Scarcity

It may be distressing
But will yield a blessing
And it will not be known
Till a day far from now

The second rune of Hagall's aett follows the theme of hardship and merciless fate. *Nauthiz* (pronounced now-theez), means "need" or "necessity." Much like Hagalaz it is a catalyst for action and personal development through life's more difficult lessons. While Hagalaz is the rune of the Norn, Urdh (past), Nauthiz relates to the Norn sister, Skuld (future). Skuld is the Norn who severs the individual's thread at the time of expiration. A fun fact about Nauthiz is that it's believed to have inspired the crossing of the index and middle fingers for good luck.

Nauthiz refers specifically to hardships of need, such as poverty, hunger, addiction, and illness. A symbol of this rune is the "need-fire," which was crucial for the survival of the ancient Northerners against the long, brutal winters. The shape of the rune resembles an unbalanced scale or the rubbing of two sticks together to start a fire. The Anglo-Saxon rune poems, which were likely written in the eighth or ninth centuries, describe Nauthiz as constrictive to the heart or chest, yet also necessary for the salvation of humans. In modern words: no pain, no gain.

In her book *Taking Up the Runes,* author Diana Paxson perfectly describes Nauthiz as "both trouble and deliverance."* The outcomes of this rune's energies are the proverbial makers or breakers in life. When we make the decision to be fortified rather than broken by struggle, we are directly working with the spirit of Nauthiz. Imagine life without difficulty. It sounds nice initially, but a life without obstacles is a life without improvement, without strengthening, without wisdom, and without appreciation for the good times. Such things are not obtained through comfort.

Additional meanings of Nauthiz include fear, impatience, survival instincts, sacrifice, limitation, and vulnerability. When life has become uncomfortable or unmanageable, we can reach out to this rune for assistance. If one finds themselves in the same predicament over and over again, they can continue to roll with it, wondering "Why me?" or they can ask, "What is this situation trying to teach me?" Nauthiz not only assists us in finding such answers but also helps us apply those answers to problem-solving. It's impossible to live a life free of obstacles, but it's possible to learn better coping skills, so when obstacles arise, we can minimize suffering. This is how Nauthiz supports alchemy of the spirit.

In readings, Nauthiz may indicate what is needed via the surrounding runes in the spread. It may be pointing out that courage and change are necessary at this time. If the querent is hoping to find out information about the future, "be patient" may be the message, especially when paired with runes like Jera or Perthro. Nauthiz warns against hasty decision-making and irrationality. It reminds us that our wants and needs are often not the same. Try not to cringe when it comes up in a reading and remember that it wants you to succeed.

When I think of the many ways Nauthiz manifests in nature, my mind instantly goes to February 2010, when the northeastern United States was hit with a massive blizzard. I remember trying to take my dog

---

*Diana Paxson, *Taking Up the Runes: A Complete Guide to Using Runes in Spells, Rituals, Divination, and Magic* (Boston, Mass.: Weiser Books, 2005), 105.

outside to do his business and the snow being three feet high. Needless to say, my eight-inch-high dachshund was not down with it. What really scared me, however, were the news stories I saw on television about ambulances being unable to make it to people who needed emergency medical attention. It was a reminder that humanity isn't in control of everything. And of course, there is our current global disaster, COVID-19. Pandemics and epidemics surely exemplify Nauthiz at its worst.

To connect with nature via Nauthiz we must leave our comfort zones (but not necessarily to the severe extent that Nauthiz tends to symbolize!). This rune challenges us to push the limits. Usually, a day of snow or heavy rain means a day inside where it's warm and dry. But what if we push ourselves out of our comfort zones and run wildly through the pouring rain barefoot? (If you haven't done this yet, I *highly* recommend it!) What if we threw on our warmest winter gear and hiked through the heavy snow? Even when we're out in the world of people and bustling life, what if we put down our umbrellas and allowed the rain to bless our bodies? Little things like this can be immensely liberating. Meditating in the rain is a favorite of mine. Of course, if the temperature is cold or if the storm is accompanied by heavy lightning, play it safe and stay indoors.

Some of you may be thinking *these things aren't uncomfortable* while others are thinking *yeah right lady, I'm not trudging through the snow if I don't have to!* These are just some of the ways I push myself to experience nature. Only you know your own limitations and what's realistic to you in the way of pushing yourself into a bit of discomfort. And who knows—you might even find that you're not uncomfortable at all! Getting myself out the door is usually the hardest part, but once I'm out running like a fool through the rain or hiking through a snowy forest, I feel a genuine sense of inner peace.

Nauthiz is a motivator and so it makes perfect sense that it's connected to Skuld, the Norn who cuts the life thread. Death is a motivator for many, and the reason for "bucket lists." If you found out you were going to die tomorrow, would you be satisfied with how you lived your life? If you found out you were going to die a year from today, would your life plans change drastically?

In his book *Dharma Punx,* author and Buddhist Noah Levine participates in an exercise called "a year to live."* Just as it sounds, the "year to live" practice invites one to live their life with intention and purpose as if they have only a single year remaining. It encourages mindfulness, a renewed relationship with life, and the tending to unfinished business, such as any amends that might need to be made.

If the process of rewilding your spirit is important to you, make time for it today. Live your life with intention and purpose. Using death as a motivator is not meant to be scary; it's meant to remind us of the impermanence of, well, everything. Impermanence is the very quality that makes life so valuable, that makes it worth living the way you want to live. Life will always have periods of Nauthiz—that's just inevitable. It will always be peppered with no-fun responsibilities and inconveniences. That's okay. So when the opportunity presents itself, run in the rain, roll in the snow, lay down in the grass, meditate under the canopy of a tree, swim in a lake, go foraging . . . do whatever reminds you that you are in and of nature, and don't forget to do it mindfully. Hail, Nauthiz!

CORRESPONDENCES OF NAUTHIZ

ELEMENT	Fire
ZODIAC	Aquarius
PLANET	Pluto
MOON PHASE	Waning
TAROT	Death
CRYSTAL	Onyx
CHAKRA	Sacral
DEITIES	Akhilandeshvari, Discordia, Eris, Fenrir, Ganesha, Kali, Set
PLANTS	Borage, Burdock, Camphor, Chicory, Gentian, Sarsaparilla

Unlike the rest of the plant and rune pairs we have discussed so far, the herbs of Nauthiz may be used as remedies for the hardships of Nauthiz,

---

*Noah Levine, *Dharma Punx: A Memoir* (San Francisco: HarperCollins, 2003), 179.

rather than herbs that represent the rune's energetics. The following plants may be invoked when bravery, strength, and resilience are needed.

Borage
(*Borago officinalis*)

"I, Borage, bring always courage" is an adage that speaks of this herb's best-known virtues: bravery and resilience. The uplifting essential oil aids in dispelling fear, anxiety, depression, or when one simply needs a pick-me-up. In her book *Northeast Medicinal Plants,* Liz Neves recommends an infusion of borage, lemon balm, linden, and hawthorn to comfort a grieving heart.* The enchanting star-shaped flowers of borage are the perfect addition to ritual baths. When it is time to step up and face life's burdens, a combination of borage and Nauthiz can help us find the inner warriors that reside within us all.

Medicinal Properties

Borage is a valuable herb for treating arthritis, convalescence, and hypertension. Its cooling demulcent qualities relieve hot and dry conditions such as fever, congestion, and inflammation, especially inflammation of the skin. The leaves are diuretic and may be used as an adrenal tonic, which helps to lift depression and treat nervous exhaustion. Borage works to decongest the lungs and purify the blood. Actions: alterative, demulcent, diaphoretic, diuretic, emollient, febrifuge, galactagogue, mild laxative, pectoral, refrigerant. Cooling and moistening. Avoid during pregnancy or while nursing. Avoid long-term use. Contraindicated for individuals with liver conditions.

Burdock Root
(*Arctium lappa*)

There's a wealth of burdock in my city neighborhood, and while I consider it to be a cleansing-ritual jackpot, most prefer to think of the plant as a pesky, invasive weed. One person's trash is another's treasure! The

---

*Liz Neves, *Northeast Medicinal Plants: Identify, Harvest, and Use 111 Wild Herbs for Health and Wellness* (Portland, Ore.: Timber Press, 2020), 140.

root may be fashioned into an amulet to provide the wearer with protection. The broad leaves, which can grow up to three feet long, are perfect for banishing rituals, as one can write upon them in detail regarding the feelings, people, or habits that need to be released.

Medicinal Properties

Burdock is a detoxifying plant traditionally used to treat fevers, liver problems, gout, and a wide variety of skin conditions. It works to gently clear the body of waste, including heavy metals. Such cleansing abilities are effective in treating acne and other skin infections. Burdock is a valued remedy for kidney stones because it works to break them down so they can be easily dispelled through the urine. It supports nutrient absorption and a healthy gallbladder. Burdock is rich in oils and targets dry conditions such as constipation. It is best used in tandem with herbs that have similar medicinal qualities. Actions: alterative, antibiotic, anticancer, antifungal, bitter, cholagogue, detoxifier, diaphoretic, diuretic, hepatic, lymphatic, nutritive. Cooling and moistening.

Camphor
(*Cinnamomum camphora*)

Camphor is not itself a plant but rather an aromatic substance extracted from the wood of certain trees. Traditionally, it has been used for incense in temple purification. It helps one to seek out and manifest their highest self. Its dreamy scent is wonderful for meditation, especially when insight is the desired result. Add the oil to a bath for auric cleansing and mind clearing. Wearing the oil can strengthen intuition and assist in rational decision-making during trying times. When a loved one dies, burn a pinch of camphor to cleanse their spirit and help guide them to the next plane of existence. As an *an*aphrodisiac camphor may be used in spells against anyone who makes unwanted sexual advances toward another.

Medicinal Properties

Some varieties of camphor are more toxic than others. White camphor is considered the safest, while brown or yellow are unsafe. Topically, it may be used as a numbing agent to soothe arthritis and back pain. Apply as a chest rub to treat congestion and cough. Camphor kills intestinal parasites. It may be used as smelling salt. Actions: analgesic, anti-inflammatory, antiseptic, antispasmodic, diaphoretic, expectorant, sedative, stimulant, vermifuge. Warming. Avoid internal use. The raw form of camphor is highly toxic. Do not use during pregnancy or with children under two years of age.

Chicory
(*Cichorium intybus*)

When I think of chicory, the Hindu deity Ganesha comes to mind. They are both considered to be removers of obstacles. They both promote positivity, attract fortune, bring success, and provide general protection. Chicory favors a good sense of humor and the ability to remain optimistic when faced with unfavorable circumstances. It was highly valued in ancient Egypt. John Michael Greer states that this plant was believed to grant the power of invisibility and magickally open locked doors.*

Medicinal Properties

A valued tonic for the liver and gastrointestinal (GI) tract, chicory stimulates appetite and aids in healthy digestion. In eastern Europe it was a traditional go-to remedy for adults and children with diarrhea. Chicory resembles dandelion in appearance as well as health benefits, in that they are both mildly diuretic, cleansing to the urinary tract, and useful in treating kidney stones. Chicory is a restorative herb that can help to speed up the process of convalescence. Decoctions have been used as mouthwash to combat tooth pain. Today, chicory is a popular salad green and substitute for coffee. Actions: bitter, cholagogue, digestive tonic, diuretic, liver tonic, laxative. Warming and drying.

Gentian
(*Gentiana lutea*)

When we suffer setbacks in life, gentian acts as a pick-me-up and helps to trade discouragement for confidence. The powdered root may be

---

*John Michael Greer, *The Encyclopedia of Natural Magic* (St. Paul, Minn.: Llewellyn, 2019), 82.

added to incense blends and burned to remove heavy energies. When comfort and emotional strength are needed, add it to a hot tea blend or bath. In cases where depression or anxiety result in lacking libido, gentian is useful in arousing sexual desire. The root is an appropriate offering to the divine when petitioning for relief from crisis.

Medicinal Properties

Gentian root is an incredibly strong bitter. The first time I took it, I followed it by shoving a chocolate bar in my mouth in an attempt to replace the intense taste of the root. It may not have the most pleasant flavor, but it's excellent for kickstarting digestion and increasing nutrient absorption. Gentian should be taken about half an hour before a heavy meal alone or as part of an aperitif. It is effective in treating anemia and heavy menstruation. Actions: alterative, antacid, antipyretic, bitter, digestive tonic. Cooling and drying. Avoid during pregnancy. Those with peptic ulcers should not use gentian.

Sarsaparilla
(*Smilax* spp.)

Sarsaparilla is a raiser of vibrations. Those dealing with illness, anxiety, melancholy, grief, or anger will find an ally in sarsaparilla. It motivates us to work hard for the things that matter to us, such as our health, happiness, and relationships. Because of its ability to raise vibrations, this perennial naturally attracts good fortune and is therefore a common addition within money and love magick. Sarsaparilla grants longevity, vitality, and a passion for life for those who have become jaded.

Medicinal Properties

Historically, sarsaparilla root was used to treat syphilis. The root is also the original flavoring of root beer. It works to purify the blood and remedies skin conditions such as psoriasis and eczema. Sarsaparilla targets arthritis, gout, colitis, and kidney disease. Actions: alterative, antibacterial, anticancer, anti-inflammatory, aphrodisiac, diuretic, estrogenic, hepatic. Warming and moistening.

11
ISA

ᛁ

Phonetic equivalent: I
Ice, Stagnation, Self-Preservation

Icicles hang like daggers
The water is now ice
We walk on treacherous grounds
Only caution will suffice

Isa (pronounced ee-sah) is the ice rune. It symbolizes delay, still-ness, cold, barriers, frustrations, and hindrances. Like Hagalaz and Nauthiz, Isa is a rune of difficulty and is associated with the Norns, specifically the middle sister, Verdandi, who is the Norn of the present. Ice is very much an element of the present, as in the past it was water and in the future it will be again.

These days ice can certainly be a nuisance but for the ancient Northerners, ice could be a matter of life and death. The frozen winters marked a time of hunger and general difficulty as the earth beneath the snow was rendered completely barren. Hunting for food yielded less due to hibernation and harsh weather. Life had to be taken day by day.

On a lighter note, Isa is a rune of rest, self-control, and homeostasis. It relates closely to the hanged man card in tarot, which has an overt connection to the story of Odin hanging from the World Tree for nine days and nine nights in exchange for the wisdom of the runes. Isa illus-

118

trates that the need for help is not a weakness but is sometimes very necessary! It's not only easier but also safer to cross over frozen ground with the help of another or with a fixed structure to hold on to. In this way, Isa may be an indication that one's current undertaking cannot be successfully accomplished without the support of others, especially if it appears in a reading alongside Mannaz.

When Isa is drawn in a reading it typically indicates that there is no possibility for change at the present time *or* that things are moving too quickly and stillness is needed. Additional meanings include the need for patience, fighting against the current, emotional "coldness," or the survival instinct. When it comes to accurate interpretations of a spread, knowledge of each rune is of course necessary, but we mustn't forget that it's intuition that will aid in discernment of nuance.

It's safe to say that Hagalaz, Nauthiz, and Isa are teachers, and that's a mild way to put it! I'm not talking about your sweet old kindergarten teacher. We know that a great teacher doesn't coddle their students—they *challenge* us; they push us to our limits and beyond. When we are overcome with fear and self-doubt, teachers help us to reach deep inside and pull out the strength we didn't know we had. In Finland they have a word for such strength, and that word is *sisu*. Sisu represents bravery and determination in the face of adversity.

Hagalaz, Nauthiz, and Isa are three no-nonsense runes that catalyze growth on microcosmic *and* macrocosmic levels within our spirits and throughout the entire cosmos. As above, so below. Isa urges us to be still and find power within before proceeding ahead. The ice rune denotes a period of quiet contemplation and preparation—a metaphorical winter that is about to give way to the welcome warmth of the coming spring.

Isa cultivates a relationship with nature through stillness. Ice pauses the flow of water, and for the ancient folk who lived in snowy regions, life itself seemed to pause with the severity of winter.

In Western society we are accustomed to fast-paced living. Everyone is on the go, trying to get from one place to the next. Like our lives, our minds are doing their own type of endless running. The introduction of meditation into Western culture has been a major lifeline as stillness and mindfulness do not come naturally to the majority. They certainly did not come naturally to me!

Meditating isn't just sitting cross-legged on the ground and chanting "Ohm." While that's one way to go about it, there are also many other ways. Meditation can be done basically anytime and anywhere. It can be done sitting on the ground, in a chair, standing up, walking, during exercise such as asana yoga, or lying down; it can be done while you do the dishes, sweep the floor, or play an instrument.

There's a misconception that meditation is synonymous with emptying the mind; I would say it's synonymous with being present. When we make a conscious effort to focus on the now, we are meditating. When we gently reel in our minds from past or future thinking and return to mindfulness, we are meditating. When we allow ourselves to experience emotions, the easy as well as the difficult ones, without resistance to discomfort, we are meditating. It truly astonished me when I realized how much pain I could save myself simply by focusing on the here and now. It sounds like such an easy concept, but like anything it takes practice.

If you've never done so before, the first time you decide to meditate probably won't go as smoothly as you'd like, and that's okay. I've been doing so for a little over a decade now and I still have sessions where I just can't seem to calm my ever-running mind and be present. Progress, not perfection.

You may have noticed by now that meditation is referenced quite a bit in this book, and that is not accidental. Let's take a quick look at the benefits of regular meditation:

- Helps rewire chaotic thinking patterns
- Improves memory, concentration, and attention span
- Reduces anxiety, stress, and stress-related conditions
- Improves sleep quality
- Improves overall mood
- Lowers blood pressure
- Enhances mental discipline

Meditation tends to get lumped into the new age category, but there's nothing new about it as the practice has been used for thousands of years. Go over the list of benefits one more time—which ones have the potential of improving your magickal practice? Your life? Probably most of them! Enhanced concentration, attention span, and mental discipline means enhanced spell work. Improved sleep, mood, and blood pressure allows us to approach magick from a state of balance, which in turn fosters a more successful outcome. When I hear someone say that they don't like meditation, what I'm really hearing is that they haven't yet found their preferred method. If this is a topic you're largely unfamiliar with, I recommend further study as it is truly foundational and can improve every area of your life. Meditation is a key practice for the witch to cultivate balance and stillness of the mind—our greatest magickal tool. Hail, Isa!

CORRESPONDENCES OF ISA

ELEMENT	Ice
ZODIAC	Pisces
PLANET	Saturn
MOON PHASE	Dark
TAROT	The Hanged Man, The Hermit, 5 of Pentacles, 4 of Swords
CRYSTAL	Aquamarine
CHAKRA	Root
DEITIES	Boreas, Cailleach, Hödr, Itztlacoliuhqui, Kuraokami, Sedna, Skadi
PLANTS	Calamint, Cinnamon, Eyebright, Ginger, Maidenhair, Myrrh, Valerian

Like Nauthiz, many of the following plants are remedial against the freezing energies of Isa and seek to establish equilibrium. Most are energetically warming plants that bring movement to stagnant situations and body systems.

Calamint
(*Calamintha officinalis*)

Calamint is lighthearted plant that helps to alleviate sorrow while promoting a genuine sense of joy. At first, I included it with the Wunjo rune, but decided on Isa when I realized that it's not only jovial but also a fighter. Lore states that calamint will drive away serpents and defeat Basilisks. It also works to defeat the sometimes drab and discouraging energies of Isa. Its sweet and aromatic qualities make it a perfect addition to teas, potions, and bath blends for the soothing of emotional pain.

Medicinal Properties

Calamint is a minty herb often used in the Mediterranean seasoning za'atar. It is diaphoretic, which means it induces perspiration—a useful quality for lowering fevers. It is a decongestant and soothing for various respiratory ailments. Calamint settles excessive flatulence and general indigestion. It treats seizure, insomnia, and depression. Calamint has a high menthol content and topically it can be applied to encourage the healing of cuts and bruises. Actions: aromatic, carminative, diaphoretic, expectorant. Cooling and drying. Avoid during pregnancy.

Cinnamon
(*Cinnamomum zeylanicum*)

Cinnamon is well known and loved for its sweet and spicy flavor. Because it is ruled by both Fire and Sun, it's an excellent remedy for the frozen blockages of Isa. Add cinnamon chips to incense or the essential oil to a diffuser to unblock the chakras—particularly third eye and root. Cinnamon's fiery energies lend themselves to love and sex magick. To awaken sexual desire, coat a red candle in oil, roll it in cinnamon and damiana, light the wick, and vibe in the seductive energies. The warming scent raises vibrations, lifts spirits, purifies and strengthens energy during spell work, and awakens the mind while aiding in psychic ability. Cinnamon is also a common ingredient in money magick and pairs nicely with the Fehu rune.

Medicinal Properties

Cinnamon is an ancient spice mentioned as far back as the Jewish Torah. Traditionally, it has been consumed to energize the nervous system, soothe a sore throat and cough, and ease various stomach issues such as gas and vomiting. It has antidiabetic actions that help to balance blood sugar levels. Cinnamon helps to speed up the process of convalescence and relieves menorrhagia. Actions: antibacterial, antidiabetic, antifungal, antimicrobial, antiseptic, aromatic, astringent, carminative, emmenagogue, stomachic, stimulant, vermifuge. Warming and drying. Direct contact to the skin via the essential oil or in baths can cause irritation or possibly burns. Ingesting excessive amounts can cause gastrointestinal distress. Avoid the essential oil during pregnancy and in any form while breastfeeding.

Eyebright
(*Euphrasia officinalis*)

When engaging in third eye or visionary work such as divination or inner journeying, eyebright is a wonderful companion. To enhance the ability of second sight, anoint the eyelids with a simple infusion or oil of eyebright. While it could work just as well with Wunjo the joy rune, or Sowilo the sun rune, I've included it with Isa because it encourages a bright outlook when life seems grim. Like the other herbs in this section, it is ideal for "melting the ice" of Isa, especially when paired with either of the main Fire runes, Sowilo or Kenaz. Bathing in eyebright helps foster clarity, cognitive strength, and peace of mind.

Medicinal Properties

Eyebright works to accomplish what its name suggests—a brightening of the eyes. It relieves seasonal allergies and itchy, watering eyes. Use as a wash or take internally for eye infections. Eyebright relieves upper respiratory infection and alleviates inner ear pain in both adults and children. Actions: antiallergenic, anti-inflammatory, antihistamine, anticatarrhal, astringent, expectorant. Cooling and drying. Do not use eyebright tinctures as eyedrops.

Ginger
(*Zingiber officinale*)

Just a small amount of ginger added to any magickal working will disperse stagnant energies and increase the power of a spell. Ginger is ruled by Mars, and it packs a punch when concentrated, forceful energy is required. Its fiery nature increases sexual desire and supports love and sex magick. As you'll see in the following paragraph, it's an incredible healer, and its benefits are just as potent in healing spells and rituals. Ginger is an excellent ally for those facing crisis or illness, as it promotes courage, vitality, and strength.

Medicinal Properties

Ayurveda refers to ginger as the "universal medicine" and recommends a small daily amount to aid in digestion and the body's ability to assimilate nutrients. It is a synergetic herb that increases the remedial potency of other herbs. Today, popular medicinal beverages that include ginger, such as golden milk or fire ciders, are consumed to increase circulation of bodily fluids, boost immunity, and reduce the risk of heart disease. Above all, ginger is best known as a digestive tonic, and relieves a wide array of issues including motion sickness, viral gastroenteritis, general indigestion, vomiting, and pregnancy-induced nausea and vomiting. It also has pain-relieving qualities that are suitable for headache and migraine, muscle pain, and menstrual cramps. As a topical, it is anti-inflammatory and may be applied as a compress for arthritic joints, sore muscles, and sciatica. The essential oil is calming, uplifting, and opens the heart chakra. Actions: analgesic, antiemetic, anti-inflammatory, antispasmodic, antiviral, aromatic, carminative, circulatory tonic, diaphoretic, digestive tonic, emmenagogue. Warming and drying.

Maidenhair
(*Adiantum capillus-veneris*)

The fronds of the maidenhair fern, also known as herbe de Freyja, encourage fiery passion and lust. The voluminous plant is a proponent of beauty and love and may be used to heat up a long-term romantic relationship that has turned cold. Maidenhair is associated with joy and is a popular plant to keep hanging inside and outside of the home. It may be used to banish harmful energies and promote renewal. Lore suggests that the seeds contain the power of invisibility. Its energies seek to purify as well as attract health and wealth.

Medicinal Properties
Maidenhair supports a healthy respiratory system and is a remedy for respiratory complaints such as bronchitis and whooping cough. It improves circulation of the blood, which improves O_2 levels in the body. As per its name, maidenhair is beneficial for conditions of the hair and scalp, especially in cases of dandruff or hair loss. It may be used to ease heavy menstruation and cramping. Actions: astringent, demulcent, mild diuretic, emetic, emmenagogue, emollient, expectorant, pectoral, stimulant, sudorific. Cooling and drying. Avoid during pregnancy.

Myrrh
(Commiphora myrrha)

Myrrh could be paired with a handful of runes, but I've included it with Isa due to its ability to remove obstacles. Myrrh breaks down dense blockages and creates movement. Its energy is gentle yet strong, perfect for those who feel that their trauma or grief will not allow them to move forward with life. When we hear of myrrh it's usually paired with its close colleague frankincense, and understandably so, as their synergy is beautifully aromatic and magickally powerful. Whether combined with other herbs or by itself, myrrh is an enchanting companion that will benefit anyone on their spiritual path. It is a powerful healer, purifier, and is ideal for blessings. Myrrh is typically burned to cleanse the energies of a space. Ancient Egyptians used it in the embalming process and today it is still valued for its use in death rites. Meditating alongside the burning incense increases wisdom and intuition. It's truly a must-have in your magickal apothecary.

Medicinal Properties
Myrrh is strongly antibacterial and works well as a topical treatment for external wounds. The resin and essential oil may be diluted and used as a mouthwash for sore throat and mouth ulcers. Add the powdered resin to blends for a natural method of treating diaper rash. Actions: antibacterial, anti-inflammatory, antiseptic, aphrodisiac, aromatic, astringent, bitter, carminative, digestive, vermifuge, vulnerary. Warming and drying. Avoid during pregnancy and nursing.

Valerian
(*Valeriana officinalis*)

Like the frozen Isa rune, valerian promotes stillness and rest as well as peace of mind and spiritual grounding. While we sleep, we are quite vulnerable, and the plant's root may be added to charms, amulets, and spell bottles for protected sleep. Valerian is a plant of healthy solitude—not to be mistaken with loneliness. Like the tarot's hermit card, it encourages periods of introspection and self-care. Due to its calming properties, a bit of the hot tea is beneficial before trance work.

Medicinal Properties

Valerian root's medicinal powers are often compared to those of the prescription drug valium. Both effectively treat stress and anxiety and encourage deep, restful sleep by relaxing the central nervous system. Actions: analgesic, antispasmodic, carminative, nervine, sedative, soporific. Due to its warming qualities, avoid in those who have "hot" constitutions. Short-term use is recommended.

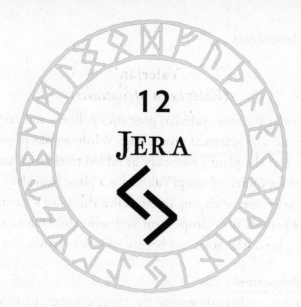

12
JERA

Phonetic equivalent: Y and J
Year, Cycle, Progress

Jera's a wheel that never stops turning
It follows the three runes of hardship and
   learning
It yields a grand harvest from seeds we have
   sown
Each season will share with us how we have
   grown

After the previous three runes, we can let out a sigh of relief with the introduction of Jera (pronounced Yair-ah), the much-awaited calm after the storm. Jera translates to year and corresponds to the letters *Y* and *J*. It symbolizes the first signs of spring after a long, bleak winter.

Natural cycles, seasons, gain, the wheel of the year, proper timing, and growth all fall under the umbrella of Jera. The wearisome winter season of Isa has finally come to pass, and the melted ice nourishes the thawed soil in preparation for sowing. The emergence of Jera brings with it the promise of liberation and opportunity.

Jera is the Earth element in action. The shape of the stave itself is indicative of what it represents—the wheel of the year, linear time, the cycles of nature, and cause and effect. If you recall, Hagalaz, Nauthiz, and Isa relate to the Norn sisters who represent the past, present, and future; therefore, the first four runes of Hagall's aett are all related to concepts of time, and Jera is a culmination of the power of the Norns.

If Jera had a slogan, it would be the age-old adage "You reap what you sow." This is certainly a rune of cause and effect. In this way we see a relation to the concept of karma. If we are unhappy with the lot life has handed us, perhaps we need to rethink the energies we put out into the world.

It's worth noting that Jera, representing the wheel of the year, is the twelfth rune in the Elder Futhark, which calls to mind the twelve months in a year. The harvest rune signifies a time of change, patience, movement, and harmony. It reminds us that there are no instantaneous results, that we must be patient and work diligently toward our goals if we wish to be rewarded or successful.

Magickally, Jera is ideal for healing, alignment, balance, and navigating the emotional and physical seasons of life. It highlights impermanence/the inevitability of change—the only constant. For those who garden, draw Jera on plant pots or in the soil of a garden bed to encourage healthy growth. I often intone this rune to my plants as well.

In readings, the presence of Jera may indicate reward, fruition, patience, the recession of difficulty, or even pregnancy. Depending on the surrounding runes, it may be suggesting where one's energies are best spent. With Fehu, the message may be to keep up the hard work as financial gain is in the near future. Paired with Ingwaz, Jera might imply that now is the time to begin that new project you've been pondering. There are no reversed or murkstave meanings.

Jera is very similar to the tarot's wheel of fortune card, which also holds the meaning of cyclical change. The world never stops turning, life never stops changing, and both Jera and the wheel of fortune card are indicative of that. As if life were a Ferris wheel, there are constant ups and downs marked by intermittent peaks and rock-bottom lows.

Jera connects us with nature via the wheel of the year, which consists of eight sabbats or fire festivals, four of which represent the solstices and equinoxes (Yule, Ostara, Litha, and Mabon) while the other four are commonly referred to as "cross quarters," which are traditional Celtic fire festivals (Imbolc, Beltane, Lughnasadh, and Samhain). Some view Samhain (pronounced sau-win) as the beginning of the pagan year, while others prefer to think of Yule as the beginning due to the "birth" of the sun—the return of longer days.

Each sabbat marks an ending and therefore a beginning. It is a time to celebrate and prepare for change. I write this chapter just before Beltane as the warming weather and constant rains yield new plant life. Beltane is the midpoint between spring and summer. The trees are waking from their deep winter sleep, and the birds are returning to my corner of the world. This is a time of year where fertility of the land and animals is celebrated, hence Easter with its rabbits and eggs.

Back in the days of old, sabbats were celebrated with community feasts, balefires, and even sacrifices to ensure that the coming season be kind and prosperous. One of the traditions of Beltane in particular is the ribbon-clad maypole around which children are known to dance. What many don't know about the maypole, however, is that it is a phallic symbol representing the fertility of the season. It is also representative of the tree of life.

Like everything in witchcraft, the eight sabbats not only reflect the changes of the Earth but also the cycles and changes within us. As within, so without. The sabbats mark periods of repose, reflection, growth, and transformation. These are periods of Earth alchemy that we can learn from and incorporate into our own spiritual alchemy. This is an excellent time for divination regarding one's current state of being, what needs to be healed, and how to go about such healing.

Each season and sabbat counsels us on how we can work the process of inner alchemy. The onset of autumn puts out the call to slow down and harvest all that has grown during the active period of summer. As the temperatures cool, death is introduced via the harvest and ending of plant life cycles. During this time, Eihwaz teaches us about the normality, and even beauty, of the process of dying. The arrival of winter brings the spirit of Earth to a halt, indicating that a period of repose and introspection is necessary. Isa can guide us through this time of stillness, teaching us the importance of healthy solitude and periodic soul-searching. As winter gives way to spring, we can call on Jera to gently aid us in turning our attention outward again. Slowly, we trade in stillness for movement. At the onset of summer, momentum increases. This is a period of high energy and passion represented by heat. Sowilo is a perfect ally for this time.

Change is inevitable, and we can choose to resist it or celebrate it. By acknowledging the wheel of the year and the eight sabbats, we are choosing the latter. If a large outdoor celebration isn't possible (or you simply don't feel like erecting a giant symbolic penis in your yard), there are much simpler ways to celebrate. Some change up the theme of their altar in line with the wheel of the year. I personally love to have outdoor fires for the sabbats, but when that isn't possible, I settle for a candle ritual to welcome the coming changes of the season. There's no right or wrong way to celebrate. Also, there's nothing wrong with not celebrating these days if you choose not to—to each their own. Hail, Jera!

CORRESPONDENCES OF JERA

ELEMENT	Earth
ZODIAC	Taurus
PLANET	Jupiter
MOON PHASE	New Moon
TAROT	Wheel of Fortune
CRYSTAL	Chrysoprase
CHAKRA	Heart
DEITIES	Chronos, Demeter, Fortuna, Ostara, Neper/Nepit, Norns, Zurvan
PLANTS	Chaparral, Hawthorn, Honeysuckle, Wild Iris, Ylang-Ylang

The corresponding plants of Jera are typically ruled by the grounding Earth element, and embody progress, reward, and the perpetual changes that we experience on both microcosmic and macrocosmic levels.

Chaparral
(*Larrea tridentada*)

Chaparral, also known as the creosote bush, was a staple of the Native Americans of the southwest United States. Spiritually, it supports personal purification, feelings of security, and favorable change. Chaparral has a fresh scent and is ideal for smoke bundles and incense. Some believe it to be the oldest plant in the world due to carbon dating. A pairing of Chaparral and Jera will help to guide one out of a spiritual (or literal) winter and into the dynamic warmth and beauty of the springtime. Chaparral and Jera help us to embrace change instead of fearing it.

Medicinal Properties

Chaparral's antiviral activity has been valued as a natural remedy against HIV. As a blood purifier it helps to treat heavy metal toxicity and radiation. This natural antibiotic can be made into a poultice or wash for skin irritations such as acne, burns, eczema, and rashes. Actions: alterative, antibacterial, anticancer, antidiabetic, antidiarrheal, antifungal, antimicrobial, antioxidant, antirheumatic, bitter, expectorant, vermifuge. Cooling and drying. Internal use should be limited due to possible damaging effects on the liver; therefore, it should be avoided by those with kidney or liver disease, as well as during pregnancy.

Hawthorn
(*Crataegus monogyna*)

Hawthorn is a tree of fertility and death, hence its utility during the Celtic festivals of Beltane and Samhain. Any part of the plant may be given as an offering when celebrating the turning of the seasons. Hawthorn aids and accompanies those who participate in spirit travel, and the thorns offer protection through unknown territory. It is ideal for all matters of the heart and helps to improve openness and honesty among loved ones. Use in spells to lessen the sting of heartbreak or grief. The hawthorn tree is sacred to the Norse god Thor. In Ireland the tree is regarded as a portal between worlds. It is ill-advised to harm or cut down a hawthorn tree, as the spirits of the land or faery folk who dwell there may have their revenge.

Medicinal Properties

Hawthorn is an amazing ally of the heart and works as a long-term tonic that nourishes and strengthens. While leaves and flowers have valuable applications, the berry is the part most used for remedial purposes. Hawthorn treats congestive heart failure, angina, atherosclerosis, irregular heartbeat, hypertension, coronary artery disease, and enlargement of the heart. The berries are high in vitamin C and improve collagen, soothe inflammation, and prevent or break down kidney stones. They contain nurturing nervine qualities and are therefore a good choice for anyone dealing with heartbreak. To reap the benefits of hawthorn, long-term use is suggested. Actions: alterative, anti-arrhythmic, antibacterial, anti-inflammatory, antioxidant, antispasmodic, astringent, cardiotonic, carminative, digestive, diuretic, mild expectorant, nervine, sedative, vasodilator, vermifuge, vulnerary. Cooling and moistening. Avoid alongside heart medications, hypotensive medications, and medications for bleeding disorders. Avoid ingesting the seeds. Hawthorn may cause allergic reactions. Avoid while pregnant or breastfeeding.

Honeysuckle
(*Lonicera caprifolium*)

The energies of honeysuckle are abundant and joyous. It helps to bring relief to those who have just undergone periods of misfortune. Those stuck in trauma or grief may find it easier to move forward and begin the healing process with the help of honeysuckle. This hardy plant reminds us that we must always put in the work and "plant the seeds" for our ourselves in order to harvest a fruitful future. The sweetly scented flowers are typically used to attract a lover. Rub the leaves or flowers between the brows to open the third eye. Combine the uplifting energies of honeysuckle and Jera when calling luck and beneficial change into your life.

Medicinal Properties

Honeysuckle combats infections of all kinds, including cold and flu, conjunctivitis, mastitis, staph, and salmonella. It has a cooling effect that aids in bringing down fevers. To soothe a sore throat, gargle tea made from the leaves. When the mind is overly nostalgic and fixated on the past, honeysuckle helps to bring one back to the present. Actions: alterative, antibiotic, anti-inflammatory, antirheumatic, diaphoretic, diuretic, expectorant, laxative, refrigerant, vulnerary. The berries are toxic, so do not ingest them.

Wild Iris
(*Iris versicolor*)

Like Jera and spring, wild iris is a plant of renewal. Also known as blue flag, this gorgeous perennial is a detoxifier of body, mind, and spirit. It helps to purge the stagnancy of winter and allow space for vitality and warmth to move in. For those with seasonal depression in winter, dried or fresh bundles should be kept in the home to promote vibrancy. The flowers attract wisdom, joy, and lightheartedness. Those who wish to reinvent themselves will benefit from the combined energies of wild iris and Jera and should call on their powers for improvement of outlook and attitude.

Medicinal Properties
Wild iris is a North American native favored by for its ability to detoxify the body via diuretic, cholagogue, and laxative properties. By detoxifying and working through the liver, wild iris aids in the treatment of skin disorders such as acne, psoriasis, eczema, and herpes. As a poultice the roots are used to soothe sores, bruises, and sprains. The scent of the root is said to deter rattlesnakes. Actions: alterative, anti-inflammatory, cholagogue, diuretic, emetic, hepatic, laxative, sialagogue, vulnerary. Cold and moistening. Somewhat toxic. Large amounts may cause vomiting. Avoid alongside weakened constitutions.

Ylang-Ylang
(*Cananga odorata*)

Ylang-ylang is perfect for spring cleaning of the mind, body, and spirit. Whether clearing cobwebs out of the house or out of the auric field, the flower's essential oil refreshes and cultivates a sense of peace. Ylang-

ylang is an aphrodisiac that represents femininity, fertility, and sexuality. The scent boosts libido and aids in fertility magick. As a flower of Venus, it promotes beauty and pleasure. To ritually welcome the spring equinox and a new beginning, use the diluted essential oil to draw the Jera symbol over the third eye, heart, and solar plexus while intoning the name of the rune. Feel the vibrations of the intonations warm and renew the energy body.

Medicinal Properties

Ylang-ylang is used primarily as an essential oil in aromatherapy. It's an advocate for heart health and helps to lower blood pressure and decrease high heart rate. The scent is ideal for soothing grief, anger, fear, anxiety, and depression. It's energizing to those afflicted with chronic fatigue. Add a few drops to skin creams or conditioner for healthy skin and hair. As an aphrodisiac, ylang-ylang increases libido and works to remedy impotence. To reap its benefits, add filtered water and a few drops of the essential oil to a diffuser. Actions: antibacterial, antioxidant, antiseptic, aphrodisiac, hypotensive, nervine, sedative. Cooling.

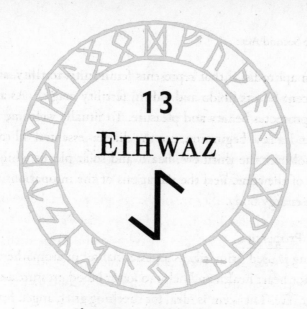

13
EIHWAZ

Phonetic equivalent: EI
Death, Rebirth, Magick

Eihwaz is polarity and the chakras in the spine
It's the twisting, winding path one walks while
*   seeking the divine*
An arrow shooting through the cosmos further than
*   the eyes can see*
And the wisdom gained by Odin while suspended
*   from the Tree*

Eihwaz, pronounced "eye-wahz," means *yew*—a coniferous tree associated with death, rebirth, and sacred ritual. Phonetically, it is the "ei" rune, although it rarely makes an appearance as a "letter" in runic writings as it is mainly used as a magickal stave.

Eihwaz is the rune of the occult. Specific to Norse mythology it refers to the mighty Yggdrasil (World Tree) and the nine worlds found within it. The World Tree is the macrocosmic representation of the human body and its line of energy along the spine. In Eastern tradition this energetic pathway includes the chakras. The shape of the Eihwaz stave is symbolic of transformation, paradox, and the twisting path to spiritual enlightenment.

As a rune of death and the occult, Eihwaz is often used within shamanic practice, astral travel, and death magick—namely necromancy. Regarding the wheel of the year, the rune relates to Samhain and provides a shield of protection when the veil is at its thinnest, repelling harmful, mischievous entities. Eihwaz is an assertive driving force, which we can see in its arrow-like appearance. It motivates us into action and helps us access the energy needed to accomplish goals. Like the previous four runes, Eihwaz illustrates the significance of change and personal development.

The serpent is related to Eihwaz. In the rune, we see the snake slithering in its shape as well as the coiled kundalini serpent that rests at the seat of the spine. As a rune of death and regeneration, it is closely associated with the ouroboros—the symbol of the circular serpent that swallows its own tail.

Eihwaz and the tarot's death card are synonymous. Both do not necessarily refer to a physical death, but rather the death of an aspect of oneself or an ending. Both the death rune and card represent the moment we stop resisting and allow immense change to take place. It's worth noting that the death card and Eihwaz are both number thirteen in their respective sequences.

While Jera represents the horizontal axes of the four elements and cardinal directions, Eihwaz is the vertical axis along which above, middle, and below reside, which represents spirit, soul, and body, or sulfur, mercury, and salt in alchemical terms. The center point where horizontal and vertical meet is the fifth element, *spirit,* and the veil between the earthly and the ethereal. It's where the atoms of our body find union with eternal spirit to create a walking, talking, thinking, and feeling human being. This point of origin is precisely why humans are always in search of *more.* We are not accepting of a solely Earth-based existence because we ourselves are not solely of the Earth.

Eihwaz helps strengthen one's connection to nature through death acceptance. In life, we deal with many kinds of deaths—some that affect us more deeply than others. Death can be a downright harrowing experience, whether it be a personal near-death experience or the passing of a loved one. Untimely and violent deaths bring their own brands of particularly traumatic energies.

While natural and inevitable, death still manages to be a source of real fear for many the world over. In the West especially, the subject borders taboo. We hand over our deceased loved ones to strangers who embalm, cremate, and/or bury them for thousands of dollars. It's always seemed very impersonal and kind of strange to me. Change seems to be happening slowly, however, especially with the rising popularity of natural burial.

Rationally we all know how our earthly journeys end, but it's the "What then?" that we struggle with most. Is it just lights out? Are we reincarnated? Does our earthly behavior determine that we are sent to either a realm of reward or punishment? Such uncertainty as well as the fear of death are inextricably tied to the concept of religion and faith. Our spiritual beliefs can provide us something concrete to hold on to within the flimsy uncertainty of afterlife.

Life itself is a series of many little deaths and rebirths. Along the way we lose loved ones as well as parts of ourselves. Like the serpent, we metaphorically shed our skins over and over again. I am not the person I was ten years ago, both on a mental and cellular level, and ten years from now I will not be the same person I am today. How beautiful that we get to renew ourselves each day, each moment if we so choose. For me witchcraft is, among many other things, exploration of the great mysteries. Almost every practitioner of magick that I know has an extensive book collection because we are seekers and *devourers* of knowledge. Death represents something that we are not yet allowed to know, and that's a bit unnerving. Some glimpse it, few even experience it and come back to resume this particular life, but until we cross over ourselves, we have no way of truly knowing.

Death magick can be incredibly liberating, and there are so many ways to go about it. One way to work with death is via the dark moon phase. Every twenty-nine and a half days the moon is not visible for a short period of time. During this lowest-energy phase of the lunar cycle, many magickal practitioners use this time for repose and reflection. Some witches altogether refuse to perform any type of magick during the dark moon.

When I began to actively acknowledge the dark moon phase, I created an altar in dedication that still stands today as one of my main altars. For the sake of balance, I keep a full moon altar as well, which stands as a celebration of life. Upon my dark moon/death altar I keep photos of deceased loved ones (including a couple of beloved celebrities who have passed, like Freddie Mercury and Layne Staley), animal bones that were found in the wild, a statuette of the goddess Kali, black candles, dried flowers, insect carcasses, graveyard dirt, and trinkets that belonged to my nanas—both of whom I was extremely close with. Hanging just above the altar is a black scrying mirror that acts as a representation of the veil that separates the realms of the living and the dead. Bodies of water (or even a small bowl of water) also work well as representations of the veil.

Reading up on the subject of death can help quell the fear, and there are some wonderful books out there on death magick, one of my favorites being *Walking the Twilight Path* by Michelle Belanger. The book is filled with exercises, meditations, and visualizations that aid in connecting to the energies of death for the purposes of death acceptance and learning to work with the other side.

When we allow ourselves to explore death in a healthy way, we provide ourselves the chance to experience nature wholly, without denying such a fundamental part of it. I believe that is what Eihwaz boils down to—a representation of the whole, the all, life and death and everything in between. It reminds us that there is no death without life, and there is no life without death. Hail, Eihwaz!

CORRESPONDENCES OF EIHWAZ

ELEMENT	All of them
ZODIAC	Scorpio, Pisces
PLANET	Pluto
MOON PHASE	Dark Moon
TAROT	Death
CRYSTAL	Nuumite
CHAKRA	Third Eye
DEITIES	Anubis, Baron Samedi, Ereshkigal, Hel, Morrigan, Oya, Thanatos
PLANTS	Chervil, Dittany of Crete, Dragon's Blood, Pennyroyal, Tansy, Yew

If one finds they've lost their way, the plants of Eihwaz may help transport them back to the center point, where they can once again achieve balance within. These plants embody the concepts of death, immortality, and magick. They prepare and accompany the traveler who journeys to the other side of the veil, where the dimensions beyond life and death may be found.

Chervil
(*Anthriscus cerefolium*)

Chervil, also known as French parsley, is one of the nine sacred herbs of the Anglo-Saxons, alongside mugwort, chamomile, and fennel. These nine plants were believed to possess special powers against all forms of malice and illness. The Anglo-Saxons believed chervil contained a powerful brain stimulant and restored the will to live in those who had all but given up. It is said to bring one to divine communion with their highest self, their infinite spirit. Chervil is associated with death and is often employed in necromancy and funereal rites. It escorts those who are leaving their earthly bodies to their unearthly destination. A basket of chervil seeds was found in the tomb of the young ancient Egyptian king Tutankhamun.

Medicinal Properties

Research on the medicinal uses of chervil so far have been minimal, but we do know that it aids in digestion, blood purification, and the lowering of blood pressure. The fluid extracted from the leaves treats inflammatory skin conditions, especially eczema and psoriasis. Actions: alterative, anti-inflammatory, antioxidant, carminative, digestive, diuretic, nutritive, vulnerary. Avoid large doses during pregnancy.

Dittany of Crete
(*Origanum dictamnus*)

Dittany of Crete is a rare find in the world of herbs, as it chiefly grows on the Greek island of Crete. For this reason, true dittany (beware of fakes online) can be a bit pricey. In ancient Greece it was a key ingredient in many perfumes, medicines, and alcoholic beverages—namely vermouth. An offering of the enchanting purple and green perennial was interpreted as a romantic gesture. It is referenced a great deal within Greek mythology. Today dittany is commonly regarded as an herb of Samhain, seance, astral travel, and necromancy. It is associated with psychopomps and underworld deities such as Hekate, Hel, Persephone, Osiris, and Anubis as well as "love" deities like Aphrodite and Venus. When seeking esoteric knowledge or invocation of a spirit, a combination of Eihwaz and dittany (especially as an incense) is a potent pair and should be used wisely and with magickal precautions.

Medicinal Properties

Historically, dittany was used to treat the common cold, digestive upsets, poisonings, venomous snake and spider bites, and to bring on menstruation. With honey, it works to soothe a sore throat and cough. It may be applied as a poultice to treat minor external wounds and draw out splinters. Dittany is soothing for menstrual cramps and headaches. Actions: antibacterial, antifungal, anti-inflammatory, antioxidant, antirheumatic, antiseptic, digestive, diuretic, emmenagogue, hypertensive, stomachic, vulnerary. Warming and moistening. Do not ingest unless under the guidance of a medical professional. Avoid during pregnancy and nursing.

Dragon's Blood
(*Daemonorops* or *Dracaena genera*)

The scarlet resin of dragon's blood amplifies any and all magick. It naturally invokes the passionate life-giving energies of fire and blood and offers authoritative protection. Burn the resin to clear away harmful energies and entities while preparing the mind and space for spell work. Due to its passionate disposition, dragon's blood works well within love and sex magick. To make an enchanted ink for bindrunes, sigil making, and writing incantations, crush one part dragon's blood resin and three parts gum arabic *or* pine sap, add enough alcohol to generously cover the powder, stir, and allow the mixture to macerate. The longer it steeps, the deeper the color of the ink will be. When ready, store in a bottle or jar and be sure to shake before use.

Medicinal Properties

Dragon's blood resin helps to heal wounds, improve circulation, treat colitis, and staunch bleeding. The resin contains antiaging and skin-healing properties. Actions: antibacterial, anti-inflammatory, antiviral, vulnerary. Neutral.

Pennyroyal
(*Mentha pulegium*)

Pennyroyal is an herb of consecration, protection, and exorcism. Greek physicians hung it in the rooms of sick patients to help clear out illness. In medieval times pennyroyal was used to repel fleas, which in turn prevented plague. It unlocks the powers and mysteries of death, immortality, and reincarnation while opening a clear channel for communication with the divine. Use as an offering when calling on spirits. Pennyroyal is said to calm chaotic feelings, especially when those feelings are triggered by the fear of death.

Medicinal Properties

Perhaps pennyroyal is best known for its ability to induce labor and terminate pregnancies. The famous nineties grunge band Nirvana even wrote a song about the heavy decision of abortion entitled "Pennyroyal Tea." This member of the mint family is traditionally known to treat general digestive upsets, as well as soothe cuts, wounds, and bug bites and repel mosquitoes. Pennyroyal calms nausea and nervous tension. Warning: Do not ingest pennyroyal for abortive purposes, as the dose that induces abortion is near lethal. Actions: abortifacient, antiseptic, antispasmodic, carminative, diaphoretic, digestive, emmenagogue, expectorant, insecticide, sedative, vermifuge. Warming and drying. Medicinally, pennyroyal should only be used by healthy adults under the supervision of a healthcare professional. Because it is an abortifacient it should be avoided by those with heavy menstrual cycles and by those who are pregnant or nursing. The essential oil is toxic.

Tansy
(*Tanacetum vulgare*)

Tansy is an herb of death, immortality, and longevity. It lends support to the recently deceased as they transition from one life to the next. It is a suitable offering to the Divine Feminine, the Virgin Mary, and within ancestral veneration. Like other Eihwaz plants, tansy assists in funereal rituals and rites, and is often used to decorate the resting place of a loved one. In terms of rebirth, it has long been a fixture of Ostara and Easter, which celebrate the resurrection of the Sun/son. Growing or hanging these perennials outside of the home is said to repel flies, rats, and demons.

Medicinal Properties

Tansy has mostly been forgotten by modern herbal practitioners, but it was widely used by cunning folk of the past for complaints such as amenorrhea, neuralgia, migraine, gas, and bloating. Applied externally, it clears up heavy bruising and relieves scabies. As a vermifuge, tansy was employed in cases of intestinal worms. Actions: bitter, carminative, emmenagogue, vermifuge. Warming. Toxic. Do not ingest unless under the guidance of a healthcare professional. Avoid during pregnancy and nursing.

Yew
(*Taxus baccata*)

The yew tree is one of the meanings of the Eihwaz rune, both of which represent death and immortality. Yews, which are often spotted in churchyards and cemeteries, can live for thousands of years. In fact, a yew tree in a churchyard in Defynnog, Wales, is believed to be the oldest tree in the United Kingdom—clocking in at around five thousand years old. There's debate on whether the World Tree, or Yggdrasil, in Norse mythology is an ash or yew. This monumental mythological tree, which serves as the axis to the cosmos, contains all the nine worlds, from Asgard (Valhalla) to Midgard (Earth) to Hel (the underworld, although not one of punishment like the Christian hell). The Norns spin, weave, and sever the threads of fate at its writhing roots. Like most plants associated with Eihwaz, yew is poisonous; therefore, the best way to work with its energies is to work with the whole tree directly. It's not advised to ingest any part of the tree, as all parts are toxic. For those lucky enough to live near one, the yew's energies may be called on for learning the mysteries of the runes, protection against malicious spirits, sabbat celebrations, and safely sending off a recently passed loved one.

Medicinal Properties
None. Highly toxic!

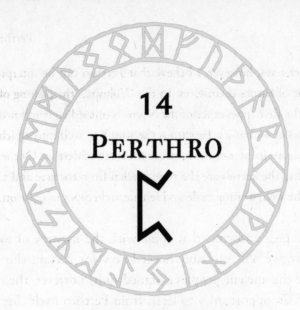

14
PERTHRO

Phonetic equivalent: P
Mystery, Chance, Birth

Perthro is a mystery
Truth hidden in the stars
Such wisdom seems so out of reach
Yet resides right where we are

Perthro (pronounced pair-thro) is a rune steeped in ambiguity and possibility. Scholars have not settled on a universally accepted interpretation, and because of the uncertainty, many have accepted *mystery* to be its meaning. With this belief in mind, its presence in a reading may be read akin to the Magic 8 Ball's *ask again later*.

The *mystery* meaning also connects Perthro to the occult, divination, and psychic ability. The shape of the rune alludes to a couple of other possibilities. Mirrored, Perthro looks like a closing parenthesis indicating an ending. Open side up it may be thought of as a dice cup, connecting it to fate, chance, games, and playfulness. Also in this position, we can relate Perthro to Ginnungagap. Open side down it resembles a squatting position suggesting the image of one giving birth. From this explanation, Perthro may be viewed as the *womb* or the *birth rune*. As author Diana Paxson so eloquently puts it:

144

At a deeper level, however, I believe that Perthro can be interpreted as the rune of Runes themselves. In the "Völuspá," the gaming of the gods and the first appearance of the Norns is immediately followed by the creation of humanity. Perthro is the womb or well into which the Yggdrasil drops its berries to stimulate the birth of destiny. One might even say that the berries are the runes, fallen from the tree and taken up from the well, uniting male and female archetypes of creation.*

There are pros and cons that come with the mystery of this rune. Unfortunately, we will probably never know for certain the original meaning that the ancient peoples assigned to it; however, the question leaves us with an opportunity to learn from Perthro itself through the process of personal gnosis. In terms of its energy, I personally tend to view Perthro as the container of all the mysteries of the cosmos, the keeper of what may also be referred to as the Akashic Records. Thus, as previously mentioned, Perthro is synonymous with Ginnungagap—the infinite void from which sprung the cataclysmic creation of the cosmos.

Through my meditations and examinations, I've come to recognize Perthro as one of the runes of the Divine Feminine alongside Berkana, Laguz, and Hagalaz. These thoughts are simply the outcome of my own exploration into the powers of Perthro, and I encourage you to sit with this mysterious rune and see what kind of energies reveal themselves to you. Pay attention to how it comes up in readings as well.

Perthro nurtures a connection to nature via the acquisition of knowledge and the investigation of natural mysteries. Witches are seekers and students of the cosmos. We are on a mission to catch a glimpse behind the veil and see how it all works—life, death, energy, will, the mind, and so on. The inclination to study metaphysics evolves from the desire to understand existence as well as our personal place within it. If you're lucky, you may have a parent, grandparent, relative, or friend who

---

*Diana Paxson, *Taking Up the Runes: A Complete Guide to Using Runes in Spells, Rituals, Divination, and Magic* (Boston, Mass.: Red Wheel/Weiser, 2005), 143.

has shown you some of the old ways. One of the benefits of social media is finding like-minded groups and individuals with whom to connect. I have made some lifelong witchy pals thanks to the World Wide Web, and I have learned so much from those friends. And then there are books. Boy, do witches love their books! So what topics can we dig into to strengthen the witch–nature bond?

I recommend starting with locality. Take time to research the plant life that grows in your area. This is a great step toward cultivating a relationship with the land on which you dwell, the genius loci, as well as the spirits of the land. There are field guides specific to location available, which are immensely helpful when you're learning about the local ecosystem. Also, if it's possible, look into your region's history on witchcraft, cunning, and paganism. Armed with this information, the modern witch is empowered through a greater connection with their environment. And with such an infinite cosmos to learn about, where better than to start with right where you are.

Of course, books aren't the only way to learn about magick. Personal gnosis is a huge part of what it means to be a witch. UPG, or unverified personal gnosis, refers to subjective experiences involving divine or spiritual revelation. Such experiences typically yield understanding or wisdom that likely couldn't have been obtained otherwise. UPG often occurs during, but is not limited to, trance, astral travel, and ritual. It was through this process that I learned the magnificent powers of Perthro.

When it does come to hitting the books, though, try to avoid doing yourself the disservice of racing through one just to get the next. I know, I know: so many witchcraft books, so little time! This is something I have done, and it often results in me completely forgetting almost everything I've just read. Take your time. Highlighting helps, and taking notes is even better. Back in college I had an anthropology professor who urged the importance of taking notes because "the average person only retains about 15 percent of the information given." That's not very much! So, make your studies count. Make it a point to put your new knowledge to the test as soon as you finish a book. Theory is useless without practical application.

Try making a ritual of the study process. Choose an appropriate astrological time to do research—waxing moons or Wednesdays are best (Wednesdays are related to knowledge and mental agility). Drink a brain-boosting herbal tea blend with herbs like gotu kola, ginkgo, lemon balm, or ashwagandha. Burn herbs that aid with focus such as rosemary, lemongrass, or tulsi. Meditate beforehand or recite an incantation similar to the one below:

> *I search for wisdom in these books*
> *Imprint their words inside of me*
> *Remember every lesson learned*
> *Retain each phrase my eyes do see*
> *By the grand power of Perthro*
> *And the sacred waxing moon*
> *I ask for mindfulness and focus*
> *I seek the knowledge of your womb*
> *Hail, Perthro!*

CORRESPONDENCES OF PERTHRO

ELEMENT	Water
ZODIAC	Cancer, Scorpio
PLANET	Moon
MOON PHASE	Dark
TAROT	The High Priestess
CRYSTAL	Labradorite
CHAKRA	Crown
DEITIES	Cerridwen, Circe, Hekate, Mímir, Saraswati
PLANTS	Amaranth, Henbane, Raspberry Leaf, Solomon's Seal, Unicorn Root, Uva Ursi

The plants of Perthro embody wisdom and esoteric knowledge. They honor the Great Mother, or Divine Feminine, and all her creations, while preparing the practitioner for profound knowledge and magick.

Amaranth
(*Amaranthus hypochondriacus*)

Amaranth is an emblem of immortality and esoteric knowledge. It provides companionship for the occult student as they seek out and explore the mysteries of the cosmos. Amaranth is an excellent offering for the Divine Feminine as well as the Greek goddesses Artemis and Demeter, to whom the plant is sacred. Historically, it played a major role in Aztec ritual practices. Because it is able to maintain such vibrancy after death, it represents the concept of eternal life and is therefore traditionally used to adorn gravesites, images of deities, and shrines. Amaranth, which means *unwithering*, lends its powers to necromancy and various kinds of spirit work. Due to its connections to spirit and femininity, it is an ideal plant for working with the *dísir*—the female guardian spirits of Norse culture. It is often employed in magick performed to repair a broken heart.

Medicinal Properties

Amaranth is valued for its astringency, which helps with excessive loss of fluids, especially in cases of heavy menstrual bleeding, hemorrhage, diarrhea, and dysentery. The leaves, which are rich in vitamins and minerals, help lower the risk of heart disease. With a high iron content, the leaves are an effective remedy for anemia. Actions: alterative, anti-inflammatory, antioxidant, astringent, diaphoretic, diuretic, emmenagogue, hemostatic, nutrient. Neutral.

Henbane
(*Hyoscyamus niger*)

Henbane, also known as poison tobacco, possesses enchanting, purple-veined flowers, a foul odor likened to rotting flesh, and is often referred to as a plant of the devil. Due to its associations with the underworld and the river Styx, it may be ritually applied to the summoning of spirits and deceased loved ones for the purpose of acquiring occult information. Henbane, which is known to enhance psychic ability, was traditionally a key ingredient in Witches' Flying Ointment along with mandrake and deadly nightshade. This endangered plant is known to conjure more than just spirits and has been employed in weather magick to bring about rain during times of drought. Historically it was used in anesthesia for its soporific effects. It is said that Henbane seeds were found within the graves of völvas.

Medicinal Properties
Due to its toxicity, henbane is no longer recommended for medicinal usage. Historically, it was predominantly used as a painkiller and seda- tive. Additional uses included treatment of heart palpitations. Actions: antioxidant, carminative, sedative, soporific. Warming and drying. For dosage information consult with a professional herbalist. Do not handle while pregnant or nursing.

Raspberry Leaf
(*Rubus idaeus*)

Raspberry leaf is a nurturing herb of the womb, and like Perthro, it contributes to fertility magick as well as workings with the Divine Feminine. This lunar herb exudes compassion and seeks to comfort those who are working through traumas, especially traumas from child- hood. As a protective charm, the leaves and berries offer safety and good health to both the expecting parent and the child. Because of its motherly disposition, raspberry leaf goes well with other feminine runes such as Laguz and Berkana. It corresponds to the Water element, cups in tarot, and the astrological signs of Cancer, Scorpio, and Pisces.

Medicinal Properties
Raspberry leaf helps to balance progesterone, prevent miscarriage, and prepare the womb for the birthing process. It diminishes nausea in early pregnancy and promotes uncomplicated labor. For those trying to become pregnant, drink a daily infusion to strengthen the uterus and prepare the body for conception. Raspberry leaf soothes irritated eyes and conjunctivitis and may be used in a gargle for mouth sores.

The berries support heart health. Actions: mild alterative, antacid, anti-diabetic, antidiarrheal, antiemetic, astringent, digestive, galactagogue, hemostatic, nutritive, refrigerant, stimulant, uterine tonic, vulnerary. Cooling and drying.

Solomon's Seal
(*Polygonatum multiflorum*)

Solomon's seal retains its name from legendary King Solomon of Hebrew lore. The king's personal seal was said to restrain demons and leave them under control of the operating magician. From its legends, we can gather that Solomon's seal is a plant of protection and warding. It aids in consecration and the procurement of occult wisdom. Cleansing one's magickal tools with this famed occult herb helps to purify, charge, and imbue the items with strong Saturnian energies. It is ideal for banishings, particularly those of sinister energies and spirits, initiation ceremonies, and the making of sacred oaths. Solomon's seal aids in manifesting the intent of the witch. To keep unwanted entities away, place bits of root near all points of entry of the home. It is also an ally for business owners who wish to ward off thieves and financial misfortune.

Medicinal Properties

Solomon's seal is a strong anti-inflammatory that helps to repair tissue damage and heal broken bones. It has an affinity for the skeletal and muscular systems. In poultice form, the root targets joint pain and swelling. Solomon's seal is one of the best herbal treatments for bone spurs. Tuberculosis, wasting conditions, rheumatoid arthritis, tendonitis, carpal tunnel, and diabetes benefit from the application of Solomon's seal. It is soothing for sore throats as well as a number of respiratory complaints. Traditional Chinese medicine regards it as a valuable heart tonic. Actions: anti-inflammatory, astringent, demulcent, mild diaphoretic, emollient, expectorant. Cooling and balancing. The berries are toxic.

Unicorn Root
(*Aletris farinosa*)

Unicorn root, also known as stargrass, is a visionary herb with a playful, childlike quality. It's perfect for those who work with mystical creatures of the astral realms, including unicorns, griffins, or the phoenix. The whimsical energy of unicorn root makes it an excellent offering for the fae folk. Also a visionary herb, unicorn root is excellent for divinatory practices, especially in the forms of scrying and cartomancy. It aids in the breaking of curses and hexes.

Medicinal Properties

Unicorn root is an estrogenic herb ideal for menstrual and menopausal symptoms. Those who have suffered multiple miscarriages will benefit from regular use while trying to conceive. It is also known to stimulate appetite and strengthen the prostate. Actions: analgesic, antispasmodic, carminative, cathartic, emetic, laxative, sedative. Toxic in large doses. Take only under the supervision of a healthcare professional.

Uva Ursi
(*Arctostaphylos uva-ursi*)

Uva ursi, also called bearberry or kinnikinnick, is a waxy evergreen shrub that is predominantly found in northern latitudes. It plays a key role in Native American spirituality and is traditionally added to ritual smoking blends. Uva ursi increases intuition, promotes psychic visions, and assists the practitioner in connecting with ancestral knowledge. Less experienced shamans have been known to smoke or drink infusions of uva ursi as they develop and hone their skills. For folks who work with bear totems it is a beneficial plant to employ when requesting their aid or general presence. The berries specifically help to cleanse and energize the sacral chakra and promote fertility. To enhance psychic ability, carve the Perthro rune on a purple or silver candle, coat it in oil, and roll it in dried uva ursi. Once the candle is prepared, light the wick, and focus on the flame while calling on Perthro to activate and strengthen psychic ability.

Medicinal Properties

The antiseptic and diuretic qualities of uva ursi benefit urogenital complaints. When taking it for urinary issues, uva ursi heals best when the urine is alkaline, so it's recommended to avoid acidic foods like cranberries (which is another natural remedy for UTIs) and meat. Uva ursi helps to prevent postbirth infections. Actions: anti-inflammatory, antiseptic, astringent, disinfectant, diuretic, laxative. Warming and drying. Not to be taken for more than one week due to strong astringency. Contraindicated in cases of kidney infection. Avoid during pregnancy and nursing. Avoid alongside kidney and liver disease as well as epilepsy.

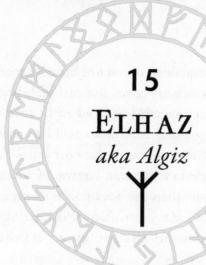

15
ELHAZ
aka Algiz

ᛉ

Phonetic equivalent: Z
Protection, Divine Support, Sanctuary

Elhaz reaches for the gods
And sings their holy praise
It will shield your heart and spirit
As it guides you on your way

Elhaz (pronounced el-hahz), the rune of protection and divine support, is arguably the most recognizable of all the runes. *Elhaz* translates to "elk" and represents defensive antlers, while the rune's other common name, *Algiz,* translates to "protection." Basic meanings include peace, sanctuary, defense, safety, and spirituality. The shape calls to mind a person reaching up to the heavens in prayer, armored antlers of an elk, or a mighty tree.

Elhaz connects us with our courage and higher spiritual selves so that we may walk our paths with a sense of safety and peace. It is the destroyer of fears, and it discourages malefic influence from drawing close. The appearance of this rune in a reading may indicate danger is close but that you are properly equipped to defend yourself. Keep your eyes open, remain alert, and trust your intuition. As with Ansuz, we must be open to incoming messages, for we never know for certain how the divine will choose to communicate. Additional reading interpretations include a time of opportunity, the need for support or protection, the need to protect someone else, a balanced relationship, or good health. Being a rune of spirituality, its presence in a reading may be informing one that their spiritual well-being needs to be prioritized.

In mythology, the protection rune corresponds to the Norse god Heimdall who resides at the Bifrost bridge between Midgard and Asgard and guards against intrusions into Asgard. He is the protector of the Aesir gods. Heimdall has impeccable sight and hearing, formidable strength, and requires almost no sleep. The Elhaz rune is the key to invoking Heimdall's level of guardianship in one's own life. A bindrune of Elhaz with Ansuz will strengthen one's relationship to Heimdall and to the divine in general. Combine with Raidho for safe journey or Uruz to support optimal health. Whatever you may need help with, the protection rune has your back.

Elhaz strengthens our connection to nature through prayer. If you're anything like me, words like *god* and *prayer* may be a bit off-putting, but let's remove the Christian connotations and consider the basic meaning of such words. Prayer is nothing more than deliberate communication with a power greater than oneself, typically where expressions of gratitude or even requests are made. The point of prayer is to build a rapport between the one praying and the power(s) on the receiving end. It can be as long and elaborate or as short and straightforward as you wish. Prayers may be offered through song, written word, meditation, or mantra.

Because I know the natural world to be a power greater than myself, I view communication with it as a form of prayer. I seek to build a relationship rather than merely having a transactional partnership, by which I mean, only giving in hopes of receiving something in return—such as aid in spell work, for example.

The foundational energies of nature—Earth, Air, Fire, and Water—are undeniably essential to a magickal practice. We can hope to raise and direct their energies simply through the use of sympathetic magick, or we can go out of our way to forge a true bond with such energies, which in turn results in some seriously amped-up magick. While this absolutely isn't the reason for having a relationship with the natural world, it's definitely a bonus! We offer prayers to deities for a number of reasons: as offerings, requests for assistance, to honor, or to simply let them know that our relationship to them is indispensable.

While Ansuz represents communication, Elhaz represents communication and the relationships specifically between humans and the divine. Deities were created out of necessity as a way for humans to make sense of nature. Before we had science to explain to us the sun, moon, stars, storms, and seasons, it all just seemed so mysterious, magickal, and intimidating. Events like eclipses and violent storms were downright foreboding. The birth of deities provided such mysteries names, faces, and characteristics—all of which were far easier to appease and form relationships with than such abstract processes and far-away celestial objects.

Making room for prayer in our lives has many benefits including peace of mind, comfort, and courage. It is therapeutic and provides us with a chance to unburden ourselves. It facilitates and reinforces a bond between the one praying and the entity being prayed to. It allows us to directly engage with the mysteries of the cosmos—that which science has yet to explain to us. Prayers of gratitude remind us that everything is temporary, and when we are consciously grateful for the blessings we have, we begin to find that we *want* less and less. When we pray to the spirit(s) of nature we are inevitably communicating with our own higher selves, as we, too, are spirits of nature. When we honor and care for nature we are honoring and caring for ourselves and vice versa. As within, so without. Hail, Elhaz!

CORRESPONDENCES OF ELHAZ

ELEMENT	All of them
ZODIAC	Aquarius
PLANET	Jupiter, Uranus
MOON PHASE	Waxing, Full
TAROT	Strength
CRYSTAL	Tiger's Eye
CHAKRA	Crown
DEITIES	All deities, Heimdall
PLANTS	Alder, Angelica, Elder, Hyssop, Nettle, Oak, Plantain, Turmeric

The plants of Elhaz are invaluable in magick regarding relationships with the divine, protection, and healing. Harmful energies are no match for this rune, especially when paired with any of the following plants.

Alder Tree
(*Alnus glutinosa*)

The alder tree is sacred in Celtic tradition because it symbolizes the balance between feminine and masculine principles. It is an excellent tree to work with when protection is needed, especially if it is believed that one is under psychic attack. Enhanced confidence and clairvoyance are supported, which in turn helps with divinatory and visionary practices. To encourage prophetic dreaming and safety during sleep, it's recommended to place a leaf inside a pillowcase. Alder, a deciduous tree, asks that we read between the lines and not take everything at face value, because there is a lesson in everything—even the mundane. As a tree of resurrection, it is fitting in rituals for the dying to send them off with protection, courage, and love.

Medicinal Properties

The leaves of the alder tree have strong anti-inflammatory qualities. Remedies made from the bark may treat arthritis, inflammation, and diarrhea. An infusion of alder may be used for sore throats, bleeding gums, and toothaches. Topical usage benefits a variety of skin conditions such as eczema, burns, and infections. Alder helps to repel insects. The essential oil soothes anxiety. Actions: anti-inflammatory, astringent, febrifuge, purgative, restorative, styptic, vulnerary.

Angelica
(*Angelica archangelica*)

Angelica's name comes from its guardian angel energies and association with the archangel Michael. The root in particular is considered apotropaic, guarding against all things evil and harmful. The powdered root may be distributed around the home to repel such things. While out and about, wearing or carrying the root provides one with a layer of protection. One of the major metaphysical applications of angelica is exorcism. To bless the home, the powdered root may be sprinkled, burned as incense, or added to an oil and used to bless every corner of the home. To purify or charge oneself with benevolent energy, add angelica to bathwater, incense blends, or make into lustral water. For those who work with bears as totem animals, it is an appropriate offering, as bears eat the roots in the springtime to kickstart their digestive systems. Angelica assists those who explore the mysteries of the cosmos and is specifically associated with the mysteries of Atlantis. In Scandinavia, the herb is sacred to the Sami people and heavily used within ceremony and medicine.

Medicinal Properties

Angelica improves blood circulation for those dealing with cold and stagnant maladies. It encourages a productive cough to relieve chest congestion. Angelica soothes indigestion, gas, and intestinal cramping. It stimulates lethargic digestion, which in turn increases appetite and bile production. Angelica is balancing to female hormones. Actions: alterative, analgesic, antibacterial, antidepressant, antiemetic, anti-inflammatory, antispasmodic, aromatic, bitter, carminative, decongestant, diaphoretic, digestive, diuretic, emmenagogue, expectorant, hepatoprotective, nervine, stimulant, stomachic, tonic. Warming and drying. Diabetics should avoid angelica. Avoid during heavy menstrual bleeding, pregnancy, or nursing. Do not take alongside anticoagulants and salicylates.

Elder
(*Sambucus canadensis*)

The elder tree has a fickle history. It is simultaneously a tree of fierce protection and one that folks of years past have desired protection *against*. The elder is said to be a witch in disguise, and it has many monikers, some of which include crone tree, tree of doom, and queen of the underworld. In England it was used to guard against lightning and protect animals from harm. Russians believed elder trees drove away malicious spirits. Sicilians employed the twigs to dispel serpents, thieves, and general mischief-makers. German lore suggested that burning a branch on Christmas Eve would expose the local witches. Throughout these examples we see the commonality of trusted protection. In many traditions the branches are hung in doorways and windows as a general means of magickal defense. Never harm or cut down an elder tree or you might find yourself cursed by the land spirits. The nickname queen of the underworld has two implications; first, it has been regarded as a portal to other worlds and second, the berries are ideal offerings for the chthonic deities and spirits of the dead. Elder trees are related to Samhain and Hel, the Norse goddess of the dead and daughter of the trickster, Loki. It is said that if one sits beside the crone tree and asks a question, the spirit of the tree will provide an answer.

Medicinal Properties

Elderberry is a prized antiviral commonly used to treat acute illnesses and support general immunity. Rich in vitamin C, it's an increasingly popular natural remedy for reducing the durations of cold and flu, especially when combined with mint and yarrow flowers. The berries have mild laxative properties. Use a blend of elder flowers and sassafras topically to reduce acne. The flowers have diaphoretic qualities, which stimulate sweating in order to relieve fevers. Actions: Berries—alterative, antiseptic, anti-inflammatory, antiviral, astringent, antioxidant, decongestant, expectorant, immunostimulant, mild laxative, nervine, nutritive. Actions: Flowers—alterative, anti-inflammatory, antispasmodic, astringent, bronchodilator, carminative, decongestant, detoxifier, diaphoretic, digestive, emetic, febrifuge, galactagogue, immunostimulant, nervine, vasodilator, vulnerary. Cooling and drying. Avoid unripe berries and fumes from the wood, as both are toxic. All parts of elder are mildly toxic and should be dried before use. Avoid while pregnant or breastfeeding.

Hyssop
(*Hyssopus officinalis*)

Hyssop is considered a holy herb, valued for its protecting and purifying qualities. It is mentioned in the Bible over a dozen times. Psalm 51:7 says,

"Cleanse me with hyssop, and I will be clean. . . ." Hyssop is my go-to bathing herb if I need to get the day's emotional yuck off me—especially after some hefty shadow work or a generally bad day. In the Middle Ages it was hung inside or strewn around the perimeter of the home to ward off plague. To remove stubborn, heavy energies from a space, the kind that just won't budge, the dried leaves may be ritually burned for exorcism; just be sure to open the windows as the smoke of hyssop is quite strong. Once the ashes from the incense have cooled, use them to draw the Elhaz rune anywhere protection is needed, yourself included. Hyssop helps to maintain peaceful vibes within the home and may be added to charms, sachets, spell bottles, and dried bundles. Add to floor and altar washes when heavy energetic cleansing is required.

Medicinal Properties

Hyssop has an affinity for respiratory health. Traditionally in the Middle East, the flowers were brewed and ingested to treat wet coughs. Hyssop helps to clear excessive mucus and relieve asthma. The antiseptic properties are helpful in treating minor wounds and bug bites. Actions: antiseptic, antiviral, carminative, decongestant, emmenagogue, expectorant, sedative. Warming and drying. The essential oil is toxic. Avoid if epileptic, pregnant, or nursing.

Nettle
(*Urtica dioica*)

Nettle, or stinging nettle, is a fiercely protective herb capable of reversing curses and returning psychic attacks to the sender. Its aggressive martial energies drive away demons, malicious spirits, and simply anyone with ill intentions. Add to baths for pre-ritual aura cleaning or to accelerate the recovery of a sick person. Traditionally, powdered nettle is sprinkled throughout and around the home for safe keeping. Baneful energies and beings are no match for nettles, especially when this herb is paired with the mighty Elhaz rune. Nettle is not one to be messed with; after all, it's not called *stinging* nettle due to its ability to give hugs! Because of its potentially dangerous yet loving energies, I often give nettles as an offering to Kali, Lilith, and Freyja.

Medicinal Properties

Herbalist David Hoffman said, "When in doubt, nettles,"* and I couldn't agree more. It's deeply nourishing, containing vitamin C, iron, magnesium, and calcium, and it is rich in protein. It helps to build healthy blood and bones. The aerial parts of the plant are great for treating seasonal allergies, especially when administered regularly in tincture form. There has been quite a bit of research done on nettles, and findings show that it significantly benefits benign prostatic hyperplasia, anemia, low blood pressure, and diabetes. It alleviates heavy menstruation, revitalizes sluggish kidneys, and speeds up the process of convalescence. Actions: alterative, anticancer, antihemorrhagic, antihistamine, anti-inflammatory, antiseptic, astringent, blood tonic, decongestant, diuretic, expectorant, galactagogue, hemostatic, hypoglycemic, hypotensive, immunostimulant, kidney tonic, nutritive, vasodilator, thyroid tonic. Neutral. When working with fresh nettles, wear gloves to avoid its irritating sting. Do not eat raw nettle leaves. Avoid while pregnant and alongside blood thinners. Because of its powerful effects on the kidneys, it's recommended to take a one-week break after three weeks of continuous use.

Oak
(*Quercus* spp.)

The majestic oak tree stands as a monument of power, wisdom, peace, protection, and healing. The shape of the Elhaz stave itself is similar to that of the armored and noble oak. Call on the power of the tree to guide you through life's trials and tribulations. Fallen branches may be brought into the home as a form of protection, and even better, they may be fashioned into the Elhaz stave with just a bit of twine. *Duir* is the Celtic name of the tree, which translates to "door," and magickally, oaks have been known to act as doors to other realms. This mighty tree is associated with Dagda, the Celtic god of wisdom, magick, strength, and fertility. For fertility magick employ acorns, as well as the Ingwaz or Berkana runes. Lore suggests that Merlin's wand was made from a branch of an oak tree.

---

*Quoted in Charis Lindrooth, "When in Doubt, Try Nettles!" BotanicWise (website), 2023.

Medicinal Properties

Throughout Europe, it was common to use oak as an antidote for poisonings. The powdered bark can be used to staunch nosebleeds, soothe ulcers, and prevent infection. A decoction of the bark effectively treats hemorrhoids due to its astringent properties. The decoction also doubles as a mouthwash for oral infections, tooth pain, and gum disease. Actions: anticancer, anti-inflammatory, antioxidant, antiseptic, astringent, diuretic, stomachic, styptic, vulnerary. Drying. Acorns should not be consumed in large amounts.

Plantain
(*Plantago major*)

Plantain is a plant of protection, especially within folk witchcraft and hoodoo traditions. It is used to repel thieves, snakes, illness, jealousy, and evil entities. While traveling, carrying the leaves helps keep one safe from malice and rough terrain. Blend with comfrey, mugwort, and/or mullein for safe-travel charms. Plantain promotes honesty and kindness. It is one of the sacred plants of the Nine Herbs Charm (which mentions Odin) in the Anglo-Saxon compilation the Lacnunga. Add to spells for healing to increase the potency of the magick.

Medicinal Properties

Plantain has a unique ability to draw out toxins and foreign material from wounds, such as splinters or stingers. This is best done by applying a poultice made from the leaves to the affected area and allowing it to dry out. A topical preparation may be used to treat hemorrhoids and ulcers. It is strengthening to the body's mucous membranes. Taken internally, plantain remedies heartburn, diarrhea, irritable bowel syndrome, gastritis, and dysentery. It is used in cases of laryngitis and inflammation of the respiratory tract. The youngest leaves offer the most nutrition and are great additions to salads. Actions: anti-inflammatory, antivenomous, astringent, decongestant, demulcent, diuretic, emollient, expectorant, mucilaginous, vulnerary. Cooling and moistening.

Turmeric
(*Curcuma longa*)

Turmeric purifies, protects, and energizes. It provides vitality and safety to the weary traveler during arduous journeys. To bless the home, sprinkle the powder throughout alongside a verbal incantation or prayer. The root may be used as a protective amulet to keep on one's person, within the home, or inside a vehicle. Add a pinch to a ritual bath to clarify the mind and aura. Turmeric's bright yellow appearance calls on the vibrant powers of the sun, and its scent is said to repel malevolent entities.

Medicinal Properties

Today, turmeric is a popular culinary spice but has long been used as a remedy for a variety of ailments such as allergies, arthritis, diabetes, gastritis, and various skin conditions. It's a valued anti-inflammatory, well suited for arthritis. It supports healthy digestion by improving intestinal flora and promoting the absorption of nutrients. Turmeric is a main ingredient in the popular ayurvedic health beverage golden milk. If you haven't tried it, I highly recommend as it's quite delicious and easy to make. Turmeric helps in the prevention of dementia, stroke, and heart attack. Traditional Chinese medicine has long valued it as a remedy for jaundice and overall liver health. The roots are rich in antioxidants. Actions: anti-inflammatory, antibacterial, anticancer, antifungal, antimutagenic, antioxidant, antiplatelet, antiseptic, aromatic, carminative, cholagogue, hepatoprotective, nootropic, stimulant, vermifuge. Warming and drying.

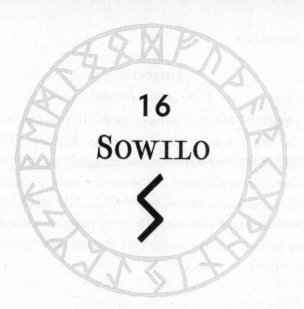

16
SOWILO

ᛋ

Phonetic equivalent: S
Sun, Higher Self, Health

Sowilo is the spark of life
The warmth on my skin
The light after darkness
The joy of my kin

Sowilo (pronounced so-wee-low) closes Hagall's aett, which began with destruction and chaos and culminates with the life source—the sun. Between Hagalaz and Sowilo, it's been quite a journey! We have survived many obstacles, learned hard-won lessons, and sought out the magick and mysteries of the cosmos only to find our higher selves waiting for us beneath the bright, warm sun.

Sowilo represents optimal health, vitality, spiritual well-being, energy, light, success, and wholeness. It is one of nine nonreversible runes. More complex meanings of the sun rune are development of the self, successfully integrating the mundane with the spiritual, and the directing of one's energy. Sowilo represents the highest force in the self, which is responsible for steering every individual's spiritual evolution.

Sowilo promotes optimism, dedication, and persistence in any endeavor. It gently exposes that which we try to hide from ourselves and others. Its warmth melts the frozen stagnancy of Isa. Magickally, Sowilo is a wonderful healing rune, especially alongside Uruz and/or Elhaz.

Many recognize the symbol of Sowilo for unfortunate reasons, as it was made infamous via Hitler's Nazi SS. Barf. Like Sowilo, the Nazis took it upon themselves to destroy the purity of the swastika, which is a historical spiritual symbol used across many cultures of the world. Some cultures, such as Hinduism, used the swastika as a symbol for the sun. While Hitler and his regimes are no longer, there's still an infestation of neo-Nazis and white supremacists that remain and attempt to corrupt these extraordinary spiritual symbols for their grossly misguided beliefs. Those of us who work with the runes and Northern traditions have a responsibility to educate others and distance these symbols from racism, sexism, and hate. Who knows, maybe someday the swastika will be removed of its contaminated meanings and restored to its true glory.

While Sowilo cannot be reversed or murkstave, like any rune it has its inimical meanings. While the sun is a source of life, it also has the ability to burn or even cause illness such as cancer. Metaphorically, this may speak of one who overemphasizes the spiritual side of the self to the detriment of the whole or balanced self. Because Sowilo represents one's highest self and/or will, adversely the rune may refer to arrogance, vanity, and even narcissism.

As a rune of pure Spirit, Sowilo enhances the connection to nature by reminding us that we are not separate from it. When the many complicated layers of humanity are stripped, we find that we are nothing more than wild animals. To some this may come as an insult, but I see it as quite the opposite. When we die what is left of us is Sowilo—our animating essence. We know that energy cannot be destroyed; thus Sowilo represents eternity.

The following is a simple ritual I like to perform every now and again, typically on a Sunday or any day when the sun is at its peak in the sky. I call it the *Onion Ritual*. Its purpose is to yield humility and remind me what I am underneath all the titles and labels I wear.

I begin the ritual fully clothed as each item of clothing will represent an aspect or layer of who I am, hence, *the onion*. Upon my altar I light a yellow, gold, or white candle in which I've carved the Sowilo rune. After a few moments of conscious slow breathing, I begin the ritual by making a descriptive statement about myself. Each statement is accompanied by the removal of an article of clothing. There is no set number or order of statements that must be made; just be sure that each one matches up with one item of clothing. That way, once you're finished speaking, you will be completely naked. The following example uses my own personal statements to give an idea of how the ritual works. Please adapt it to include the titles that are relevant to you.

"I am a business owner." As I say this aloud, I remove one shoe. Through my action and words, I symbolically remove that aspect of myself.

"I am a writer." I remove the other shoe.

"I am a neighbor." Then one sock.

"I am a friend." And the other.

"I am a daughter." I remove my hat.

"I am a mother." I remove my pants.

"I am a witch." I remove my shirt.

"I am a woman." I take off my bra.

"I am a human." Finally, I remove my underwear.

Once I am completely naked, I state: "I am energy. I am eternal spirit. When my physical body has gone, Sowilo remains." At this point I continue to stand while maintaining eye contact with the flame, which represents my highest self. I envision and feel the flame in my center near my heart. With my mind's eye I "see" the fire glowing inside of me and "feel" its heat circulating through my body and pervading my aura.

The ritual ends in silent reflection or meditation. When I am finished, I thank Sowilo and my highest self and extinguish the candle. Sometimes I will keep the vibe going and take a ritual purifying bath, or I may simply get re-dressed and continue on with my day. Hail, Sowilo!

CORRESPONDENCES OF SOWILO

ELEMENT	Fire
ZODIAC	Leo
PLANET	Sun
MOON PHASE	Full
TAROT	The Sun
CRYSTAL	Sunstone
CHAKRA	Crown
DEITIES	Amaterasu, Apollo, Baldur, Lugh, Ra, Sol, Surya
PLANTS	Calendula, Fenugreek, Goldenrod, Reishi, Saffron, St. John's Wort

The plants of Sowilo harness the power of the Sun—powers of vitality, light, success, and joy. Sun energies are often associated with abundance and work well with the Fehu rune as well. Apply the following plants to magickal workings of joy, health, career, money, and spiritual growth.

Calendula
(*Calendula officinalis*)

Also commonly referred to as pot marigold, the lovely calendula imparts energies of warmth, light, and optimism. It is one of my favorite flowers to bathe in due to its talent for purifying the aura and calming the physical body. I find this is especially effective when combined with hyssop, lavender, and a bit of sea salt. Because I live in Pittsburgh, where sunshine can be a rarity during certain times of year, I love to add calendula to teas and body oils when a boost of solar energy is needed. Calendula supports legal justice, job success, and general healing. It has associations to the Norse goddess Freyja and her prized golden necklace, the Brísingamen. Calendula lends its powers to love and passion; to promote a healthy libido, sprinkle petals around, or even on, the bed. Added to bouquets and garlands it will bless a couple with love and luck during a handfasting ceremony. In Mexico, calendula and true marigold (*Tagetes* spp.) are used to bring joy and decorative adornments to the graves of passed loved ones.

Medicinal Properties

Calendula is a wonderful topical remedy for a multitude of skin conditions such as eczema, cuts, bruises, burns, big bites, fungal infections, and hemorrhoids. When applied to superficial or deep wounds it helps to staunch bleeding, relieve inflammation, and prevent infection. This warming flower's diaphoretic properties target deep fevers that are usually accompanied by body aches. When paired with ginger, it makes an effective medicine for gastrointestinal distress such as colitis. Calendula, chamomile, lavender, and rose may be infused into a post-bath oil for infants—a blend that also aids in the relief or prevention of diaper rash. Being mildly estrogenic, it may help ease the discomfort of menstruation. Actions: antibacterial, anti-inflammatory, antiseptic, antispasmodic, antiviral, astringent, detoxifier, diaphoretic, vulnerary. Cooling and drying. Avoid internal use during pregnancy.

Fenugreek
(*Trigonella foenum-graecum*)

Fenugreek is associated with the Greek sun god, Apollo, and can be used to invoke any solar deity of your choosing. As an herb of increase and luck it has traditionally been applied to spells for wisdom, fertility, and wealth. Add to recipes, incense blends, or simply leave it as an offering during Litha celebrations when the sun is at its peak. Fenugreek is said to promote healthy decision-making, and thus would have been extremely helpful to me in my twenties! To gain wisdom, sip an infusion of fenugreek tea and call on Sowilo to unveil the knowledge of your highest self. Don't forget to offer words of gratitude in return.

Medicinal Properties
Fenugreek is a restorative following illness, and is valued within ayurvedic, Greek, and traditional Chinese medicine systems. It promotes weight gain, especially for those recovering from eating disorders. Fenugreek balances blood sugar levels and lowers cholesterol. Topical formulations work well for dandruff, sores, and burns. In ancient Egypt, the seeds were used to induce labor, and today they are commonly used to encourage the production of breastmilk. Actions: antidiabetic, anti-inflammatory, decongestant, detoxifier, emollient, expectorant, febrifuge, galactagogue, laxative, mucilaginous, vulnerary. Warming and drying. Avoid during pregnancy.

Goldenrod
(*Solidago virgaurea*)

Goldenrod is an herb of Solstice celebrations and rites honoring the Sun. It supports divinatory practices by encouraging the gifts of prophecy and clarity. It is said that a stalk of goldenrod may be used as a dowsing rod to aid one in finding a place or lost object—something I should consider trying since I lose things like it's my job, and I also have zero sense of direction, but hey, enough about my minor shortcomings. Taken as tea, goldenrod aids one in becoming more attuned with psychic ability.

Everyone's got it; some just need a bit of extra help to activate it. With an infused oil made from this vibrant plant, draw the Sowilo rune over the heart to encourage joy, compassion, and gratitude. Goldenrod is an ally for working with and clearing the solar plexus chakra. Plant the sunny herb near your front door to attract money, peace, love, and prosperity for all who dwell in the home.

Medicinal Properties

Goldenrod supports urinary health and responds to obstructions, infections, and inflammation. It is one of the best herbs to use for the passing of kidney stones. It treats congestion, sore throats, seasonal and feline allergies, respiratory infections, and yeast infections. Apply as a topical for sore muscles, arthritis, or carpal tunnel. Goldenrod eases diarrhea and gastroenteritis, especially in children. Actions: antifungal, anti-inflammatory, antioxidant, antiseptic, aromatic, astringent, carminative, diuretic, kidney tonic, stimulant, vulnerary. Warming and drying. Avoid during pregnancy and nursing. Those with kidney disease should not take goldenrod. Take extra precaution when foraging goldenrod, as it has many lookalikes, some of which are deadly.

Reishi
(*Ganoderma lucidum*)

While not "magick" in the sense of *psychedelic,* reishi is certainly a magick mushroom any way you slice it! The Chinese name is *lingzhi,* which translates to "mushroom of immortality." It helps one to make sense of the more difficult times in life, such as loss of income, break-ups, or the death of a loved one, by revealing wisdom and silver linings. Reishi promotes mental clarity and an overall sense of peace, therefore making it a wonderful ally for meditation. Like the sun it can reveal one's source of power and grant access to higher consciousness.

Medicinal Properties

The rest of the world is beginning to get on board with what Eastern medicine traditions have known for thousands of years: those mushrooms are nothing short of miraculous! Reishi has been used as a remedy for millennia and is an incredible healer. It is considered an adaptogen, which is a natural substance that adapts to what the body needs, resists damage caused by stress, and promotes overall balance; basically, adaptogens are superhero plants! A tonic made from the extract supports brain and heart function, improves sleep, relaxes muscles, reduces cholesterol, soothes chronic pain, relieves allergies, treats altitude sickness, and helps to prevent cancer. Traditional Chinese medicine cites it as a tonic of vital energy or *chi*. For animals with cancer, autoimmune disease, allergies, nervousness, and depletion, among other things, reishi is an excellent supplement. Actions: adaptogen, alterative, anti-allergenic, antibacterial, anticancer, anti-inflammatory, antioxidant, antiviral, expectorant, cardiotonic, hepatoprotective, immunostimulant, nervine, nutritive, tonic. Warming and balancing. Use caution alongside anticoagulants.

Saffron
(*Crocus sativus*)

Saffron is an herb of good health, vitality, and clarity of the mind. To enhance focus of the mind and open the third eye, take as a tea; this is particularly helpful before magick and divination. It may be burned as incense while performing healing rituals or added to jewelry charms to protect the wearer from illness. Saffron works to take the edge off depression while simultaneously providing motivation. It's said that adding it to the washer with bed sheets and clothing will increase a person's health and physical strength. As an aphrodisiac, it is a perfect addition to love potions as it provides sexual energy and a radiant shade of red.

Medicinal Properties

Saffron is one the best anti-inflammatory herbs available. It is quite pricey, but a little goes a long way. The bright red stigmas of the flower are ideal for treating depression and trauma. Saffron supports eye health, cognitive function, and memory and reduces the severity of PMS and cramps. Actions: antidepressant, anti-inflammatory, antispasmodic, aphrodisiac, carminative, diaphoretic, emmenagogue, neuroprotective, nootropic, stomach tonic. Warming and drying.

St. John's Wort
(*Hypericum perforatum*)

Fuga daemonum is an ancient moniker of St. John's wort and translates to "scare devil," suggesting its use as an herb of exorcism. Its Yiddish name, *shudim shuts,* echoes the same belief in its translation "demon protection." St. John's wort is ruled by the sunny sign of Leo and targets healing within the solar plexus. It alleviates depression and mental unrest and is often used in workings for mental health. As an herb of Fire, it's beneficial for communicating with fire elementals, which are known as salamanders. It protects against mischievous faeries and spirits. Due to its unpleasant aroma, it is more often used as a strewing herb opposed to incense. Hang the flowers above the entrances of the home to ward off bad storms, lightning, fires, curses, and demons. Lore states that St. John's wort is at its highest magickal potency during the summer solstice, or Litha.

Medicinal Properties

St. John's wort is a popular herbal treatment for all levels of depression and anxiety. In ancient Greece, it was used to treat psychotic episodes. This versatile nervine soothes fear, nerve pain, and nerve damage. It helps those who suffer from insomnia find relief. St. John's wort regulates digestion and increases appetite. The herb's strong antiviral activity treats influenza, herpes, shingles, mononucleosis, and hepatitis B and C. The tea aids in calming an overactive bladder. As suggested by its Latin name *perforatum,* St. John's wort is valuable in the treatment of puncture wounds as it heals deep into the dermis, the inner layer of skin. It helps to prevent blood poisoning such as tetanus. Folk healers in eastern Europe valued it as a remedy for kidney and intestinal complaints. Actions: antidepressant, antiseptic, antiviral, digestive tonic, nervine, vulnerary. Cooling and drying. Large doses may cause photosensitivity in those with fair skin. Avoid alongside SSRI medications. Avoid while pregnant or breastfeeding.

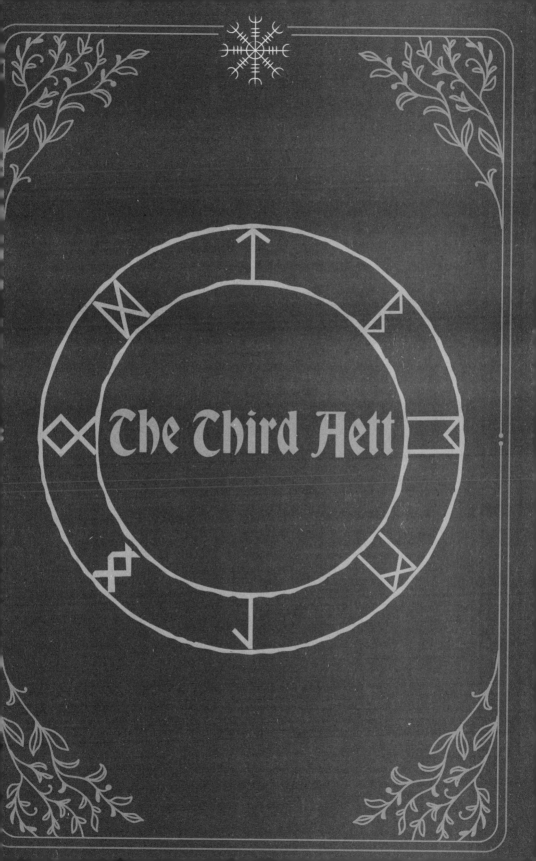

The Third Aett

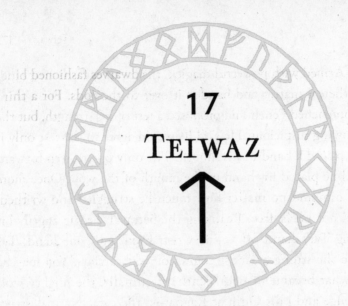

17
TEIWAZ

↑

Phonetic equivalent: T
Victory, Sacrifice, Justice

It was a sacrifice for all
When Fenrir took the hand
From the gallant sky god Tyr
The bravest fighter in the land

Teiwaz (pronounced tee-wahz) inaugurates the third and final aett, called Tyr's aett, named for the one-handed sky god to whom the rune is associated. The tale of how Tyr lost his hand is one of the more famous tales within Norse mythology.

The fierce Fenrir wolf, son of Loki, was growing more massive and mighty every day. The gods took notice of such ferocity and worried Fenrir may become a danger to them, so they devised a plan. They asked Fenrir if they could bind him in chains to test his strength, but in reality, they desired to keep him bound. Fenrir agreed, and as soon as they chained him, he effortlessly and proudly broke through. The gods cheered with praise but secretly they were disappointed. Soon the gods returned to Fenrir with stronger fetters and asked if they could bind him once more. He agreed and again broke through the fetters with ease. The gods knew they had to step up their game, so they approached the crafty dwarves of Svartalfheim to create the strongest bindings in the cosmos. Armed with powerful magick, the dwarves fashioned bindings from ethereal matter and handed it over to the gods. For a third time they approached Fenrir and proposed a test of his strength, but the wolf was growing suspicious. He said he would agree to the test only if one of gods placed a hand in his mouth. The only one to step forward was Tyr, and he placed his hand in the mouth of the wolf. Once more they bound him and no matter how much he struggled and writhed, Fenrir could not break free. Realizing the betrayal, Fenrir angrily bit down, taking Tyr's hand off at the wrist. Even with one hand, Tyr proved to be the strongest, most courageous of warriors. You may be wondering what became of poor Fenrir? Eventually, the mighty wolf gets his revenge and kills Odin at Ragnarök, the cataclysmic destruction of existence.

Even for those unfamiliar with Norse mythology, Odin, Thor, and Loki are recognizable names thanks to movies and comic books. Tyr on the other hand (pun intended) is a lesser-known god; however, you reference him once a week whether you realize it or not. Tyr, also known as Tiw, is the root of the English word Tuesday. He is the Norse equivalent of the Roman god Mars, hence why Tuesdays are ruled by the planet Mars. That's why in French the word for Tuesday is *Mardi* and in Italian it's *Martedi*. Pretty cool, right?

The Teiwaz rune represents sacrifice just as Tyr sacrificed his hand for the safety of the gods. It is a rune of masculine sexual energy, law and order, honor, and courage. Magickally, this rune will help one gain justice as long as they have right on their side.

In readings, Teiwaz typically indicates victory. It may also point out the need for courage, objectivity, or fairness. Alongside Berkana, Tyr's rune represents duality and balance. If it appears in a reading next to Raidho it may indicate the need to step up and take control or responsibility for a situation. Teiwaz is associated with the ability to handle conflicts intelligently and honorably. It was said that if a warrior carved this rune on their weapon, they would always emerge victorious from battle. Murkstave meanings include futility, misapplication of warrior energy, loss of passion, cowardice, or injustice.

Teiwaz helps us connect to nature by way of the Divine Masculine.

Before I continue, I want to make clear that the concepts of the Divine Masculine and Feminine in no way negate gender fluidity. Gender is a spectrum—masculine and feminine being the polar opposites of each end. Between the two are many shades of gray, and regardless of how one was born or how they identify, everyone has a mix of both Divine Feminine and Divine Masculine qualities. What's different from person to person are the ratios. Swiss psychologist Carl Jung referred to these gender aspects as anima (female characteristics) and animus (male characteristics).

Whether we identify as female, male, or nonbinary, we can all work with and honor the Divine Masculine within us. As someone who has identified as a feminist since a very young age, working with my Divine Masculine was not a concept that came easily at first. In feminism, we seek *equality,* a term synonymous to words like *neutral, fairness,* and *balance.* It took me some time to understand that if we are striving for a world where women and nonbinary people are in balance with men, then we must first create such a balance within the self.

So, what exactly *is* Divine Masculinity? In short, it is a variety of cosmic energies that include action, strength, movement, intellect, courage, desire, fatherhood, and the sun. You may recognize many of these facets from Teiwaz and its patron god, Tyr. It is represented as yang in the Chinese yin-yang symbol. To work with our own Divine Masculine is to acknowledge and honor these aspects within ourselves as well as within nature.

For some, working with the masculine part of the self means exploring and healing the feelings and beliefs we have toward fatherhood or manhood in general. Masculinity is not synonymous with *toxic* masculinity or patriarchal values.

I have found that, for me, the best way to honor this part of myself (and this part of all of existence, really) is through my relationship with the Egyptian deity Thoth. Of the four main deities with which I have relationships, Thoth is the only male (not for any particular reason, that's just how it happened). If you work with any gods, this might be a good place to start in incorporating the Divine Masculine into your practice and life as a whole.

If you don't have a patron deity, that's totally fine; some folks have *fulltrúis* (friendships) with deities that are more casual, but like any friendship, love and trust are imperative. Some, like me, do not view deities as sentient beings at all and merely work with their *archetypes,* which means to work with the specific characteristics and energies of them. Like Odin and Hermes, Thoth is an archetype of the intellectual and the messenger. He is the god of language, writing, wisdom, occult knowledge, art, magick, and the moon. He is the creator of hieroglyphics, which are essentially runes in their own right.

Whether it's a god that you have a relationship with or one that you simply enjoy based on their mythology, learning their characteristics and importance in lore can act as a gateway into the exploration of the Divine Masculine. If you're not sure which god to include in your exploration, Tyr is an excellent option as his characteristics are almost identical to the concept of the animus. Below you'll find a short list of deities from various cultures who, like Tyr, fit the warrior archetype. Hail, Teiwaz!

CORRESPONDENCES OF TEIWAZ

ELEMENT	Air
ZODIAC	Capricorn
PLANET	Mars
MOON PHASE	Waxing
TAROT	Justice
CRYSTAL	Bloodstone
CHAKRA	Root
DEITIES	Athena, Chiyou, Cú Chulainn, Durga, Horus, Mars, Tyr
PLANTS	Aconite, Celandine, Fig, Galangal, High John the Conqueror, Poplar, Wood Betony

The plants of Teiwaz embody the strength of a warrior and represent triumph, bravery, and male virility. The following plants are valuable in workings for justice or when courage is needed.

Aconite
(*Aconitum* spp.)

Famous herbalist and horticulturist Mrs. Grieve calls aconite "one of the most formidable poisons which have yet been discovered."* Aconite, which is called Tyr's Helm in northern Europe, was used to poison arrowheads in an effort to create more dangerous weapons. It was sometimes an ingredient of the legendary Witches' Flying Ointment, which was used to alter states of consciousness and allow witches to "fly" through the blend's psychotropic properties. Aconite, however, was a questionable ingredient because not only is it highly poisonous, it's also non-hallucinogenic and noneuphoric. It is well known by the nickname *wolfsbane* due to its purported magickal ability to cure were-wolves and its not-so-magical ability to kill wolves. The root of the plant is associated with the "angel of death," also known as a *reaper,* and has a history of being burned at funerals. As a chthonic plant, it is linked with Hekate, the Greek triple goddess of the crossroads, and her three-headed hound Cerberus, whose venomous saliva ran laced with the plant's poison. Traditionally, aconite has been utilized for cauldron, athame, and dagger consecrations. It offers protection against attack by vampire or werewolf, as well as from harmful energies during veil-crossings and death rituals.

Medicinal Properties
None. Highly toxic!

Celandine
(*Chelidonium majus*)

Greater celandine, not to be confused with lesser celandine, invokes the ferocity of the mighty Fenrir wolf by supporting one in breaking the bonds put in place by past traumas. The energies of this herb are rebellious and dignified. It helps to expose lies, mistreatments, and megalomania. Celandine is anarchic, associated with repelling law enforcement officers and corrupt authorities. It lends its powers to spells for gaining legal justice and releasing the wrongfully imprisoned.

*Maud Grieve, "Aconite," Botanical.com, 2021.

It is valued as a visionary herb and is associated with the Celtic sabbat of Imbolc. Call on the powers of Teiwaz and celandine to expose the malicious intent and actions of others and bring justice where it's due.

Medicinal Properties

Celandine covers a wide variety of complaints, especially those of the digestive system, liver, gallbladder, and eyes. It treats respiratory illnesses including bronchitis, asthma, and whooping cough. Those with warts, ringworm, and eczema may benefit from a topical preparation made from celandine. Historically, it was used to treat jaundice and liver disease. Actions: alterative, antibacterial, anticancer, antifungal, anti-inflammatory, antispasmodic, antiviral, bitter, cholagogue, diaphoretic, diuretic, emetic, expectorant, laxative, liver tonic, vulnerary. Cooling. While Celandine was a popular medicinal herb in the past, its popularity has decreased due to its toxic effects. It should only be used under the supervision of a healthcare professional. It should especially be avoided by children and people with liver disease and heart problems. Avoid during pregnancy and nursing.

Fig
(*Ficus carica*)

In ancient Greece, Spartan athletes and warriors ate figs to improve stamina, as well as to encourage bravery and wisdom. As with any plant that produces plenty of seeds, the fig is associated with fertility, especially regarding male potency and virility. *A Compendium of Herbal Magick* by Paul Beyerl suggests its utility for those who work with wolves as a totem animal. Figs make the perfect offerings for any of the gods of the Greek and Roman pantheons, but also to the god Tyr, because like him, they represent courage, working with wolves, and male fertility. It is worth noting that the Buddha attained enlightenment beneath a fig tree called the Bodhi tree.

Medicinal Properties

Figs promote digestive health and relieve constipation due to their high fiber content. Research has found that they are potentially anticancer and supportive of cardiac health. Actions: analgesic, aphrodisiac, digestive, emollient, expectorant, laxative, nutritive. Warming and moistening. The latex, a milky substance within figs, is mildly toxic, do not ingest.*

Galangal
(*Alpinia galanga*)

Galangal, also called Low John, is a member of the ginger family. Like its relative, it brings the power of Fire to any formulation or spell work. When courage is needed, carve the Teiwaz rune on a piece of the root, which may then be chewed or kept on one's person. Galangal is a warming sexual stimulant; to reap its benefits as an aphrodisiac, ingest as a tea or add a pinch of the powder to massage oil. Like Teiwaz, galangal helps the bearer obtain legal justice during court battles as long as right is on their side.

Medicinal Properties

The benefits of galangal root are many, but like its relative ginger, it is perhaps best known for a remarkable ability to settle gastric complaints such as diarrhea, hiccups, motion sickness, and vomiting. This Southeast-Asian native supports brain health by working to lessen cognitive degeneration as one ages. It works to reduce the symptoms of osteoarthritis. This warming plant soothes colds, flu, asthma, and other respiratory ailments. It fights fungal and bacterial infections. Actions: antibacterial, anticancer, antiemetic, anti-inflammatory, antifungal, antioxidant, aphrodisiac, carminative, digestive, expectorant, nervine, stimulant. Hot and drying. Avoid while pregnant or nursing.

High John the Conqueror
(*Ipomoea jalapa*)

We've just met Low John; now it's time to meet High John, also known as High John the Conqueror. Both roots are staples in hoodoo and root work. Like Low John, it is beneficial in matters of legal justice. For those

---

*SaVanna Shoemaker, "All You Need to Know about Figs." *Healthline* (website), June 3, 2020.

seeking legal victory, lore recommends chewing a piece of the root and spitting the juice on the courtroom floor before the judge takes their seat. I'm going to have to disagree with the spitting part, however, as I can't see that going over well with the judge! High John oil is often used to dress candles, as well as anoint crystals, talismans, and other tools of the trade. Its energies promote abundance, courage, sexuality, and the ability to overcome obstacles. Combine with mint and other money-attracting herbs to increase cash flow. If a curse or hex is believed to have been placed on the home, High John the Conqueror may be added to a floor wash or incense blend to remove the harmful energies.

Medicinal Properties
Toxic. Do not ingest.

Poplar
(*Populus* spp.)

As a tree of valor and perseverance, poplar wood is an excellent choice for wands. In one of the Greek myths, the god Hades falls in love with a beautiful nymph named Leuce, whom he takes to the underworld where she'll be by his side. Eventually Leuce dies and Hades transforms her into a poplar tree in the Elysian fields so she may continue to live on. This story illustrates one of poplar's most common magickal uses, which is honoring the dead. The tree's power aids in inducing clairvoyance, which is achieved by dabbing a poultice of the leaves between the brows where the third eye resides.

Medicinal Properties
Poplar buds treat respiratory complaints, reduce fever, and relieve gout. They support digestion as well as kidney and liver function. A topical poultice made from the bark soothes burns, wounds, and rashes. All parts of the tree fight pain, diarrhea, seasonal allergies, cold, and flu. It is said to aid in the drying of breastmilk when the baby is weaned from the breast. Actions: alterative, analgesic, anti-inflammatory, bitter, diuretic, pectoral. Cold.

Wood Betony
(*Betonica/Stachys officinalis*)

Wood betony is an herbal ally for those seeking justice, especially in cases of sexual abuse. It comes in handy when casting sacred space due to its strong cleansing and protecting qualities. Adding to a bath promotes cleansing and protection to the auric field. Keep wood betony near the bed or in a pillowcase to ward off bad dreams. Give as an offering when attempting to contact the spirits of the land. The Anglo-Saxons wore wood betony as charms to provide a constant shield of protection.

Medicinal Properties

Wood betony helps to relax muscles, strengthen nerves, and calm the anxious mind. The herb is often combined with other nervines to increase effectiveness. It is a common remedy for heartburn, insomnia, diarrhea, back pain, facial pain, neuralgia, muscle tension, and chronic headaches. The leaves are purifying to the blood. Wood betony calms excessive sexual energy. Actions: analgesic, antibacterial, antioxidant, antispasmodic, astringent, bitter, circulatory stimulant, nervine, sedative, sternutatory, vulnerary. Cooling. Large doses may cause vomiting. Avoid during pregnancy.

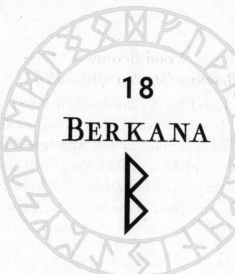

18
BERKANA

Phonetic equivalent: B
Birth, Mother, Nurturing

The divine mother tree
Is protective of me
I take shelter beneath
Her green canopy

We entered the final aett with the aggressive masculine energy of Teiwaz, rune of the sky god Tyr. Now we move to the other end of the spectrum to Berkana (pronounced bear-kah-nah) the nurturing Earth mother and goddess. In the mother rune we find sanctuary, protection, wisdom, and the tough love we all need every now and again.

The meaning of *Berkana* is "birch," a tree associated with beginnings and birth. The shape of the Berkana stave is likened to the swollen belly and breasts of a pregnant woman, thus it is a representative of sacred fragility. If you open the center diagonal lines of the stave, the shape becomes Perthro—the womb. In chapter 14 I noted that if you turn the rune of fate on its side, it resembles one in a squatting position, which is often used during the birthing process. Berkana is the mother and Perthro is the womb within that contains all. One cannot exist without the other. As a bindrune, the two symbolize the pinnacle of feminine magick—add Hagalaz and Laguz to the mix and that energy becomes absolutely earth-shattering!

Berkana provides fertile ground for new ideas and life ventures. With its creative and emotional energies, the mother rune is the perfect ally for artists and creators of all kinds. Its goddess energy is evocative of Freyja, Frigga, and the dísir. Because it is a rune of motherhood it identifies with Frigga, the wife of Odin and mother of Baldur, Hermod, and Tyr. Some believe that Freyja and Frigga are one and the same.

Call on Berkana to increase compassion and empathy or to simply assist in honoring the Divine Feminine within. It supports those who are healing from traumas such as sexual assault, harassment, miscarriage, or stillbirth. The birch rune is ideal for rituals of fertility, the moon, childbirth, rites of passage, and protection for parents and children. Because of the tree's associations with beginnings and Mother Earth, it is one of the best woods to use in rune-making.

I have a special bond with Berkana. It is the first rune I ever pulled, and as someone who has always strongly identified with the nurturing mother archetype, even before I had a child of my own, I found it to be quite profound. It was as if the runes said to me "We know you. Now it's time you know us." After that I dove headfirst into a relationship with the Elder Futhark, and I never looked back.

In a reading Berkana may be viewed as the emergence of a new chapter, especially if it follows transformational runes such as Eihwaz or Dagaz. The mother rune also brings messages of growth, nurturing, compassion, and literal parenthood. In readings regarding career, Berkana may be pointing to specific skills that should be nurtured and honed. Alongside runes of health like Uruz or Sowilo, Berkana brings the message of the importance of self-care and healthy habits. *Patience* is another key term here as we know it takes time for good things to come to fruition, as in pregnancy or the journey from seedling to tree. Murkstave, the mother rune may indicate sterility, insecurity, stunted growth, loss of creativity, endings, and apathy.

Through the power of the Divine Feminine, Berkana strengthens the connection to nature. Consider some of the monikers of our planet:

Mother Earth, Mother Nature, and Gaia—the Greek personification of the Earth and mother to all life on it.

Whether we identify as female, nonbinary, or male, we can celebrate the Divine Feminine and the anima within us all. Like the Divine Masculine, the Divine Feminine is composed of a variety of cosmic energies, which include life-giving, sensitivity, receptiveness, sensuality, intuition, and motherhood. It is represented as yin in the Chinese yin/yang symbol. To work with our own divine femininity is to acknowledge and honor such aspects of ourselves no matter how we identify.

The mother archetype is exhibited in all mythologies and cultures, and I have listed a handful of them in the following correspondence section. Whether you choose to work with the Divine Feminine in the form of a deity is entirely up to you. For those who incorporate the triple moon concept into their practice, which consists of maiden (waxing phase), mother (full moon), and crone (waning phase), the full moon is a truly auspicious time to activate and align with the mother archetype. (Notice how the moon's magickal energies are almost identical to that of the anima. We see the same correlations between the sun and the animus.) No matter your gender or parental status, you contain within yourself the anima, the mother archetype, and the Divine Feminine; below we will explore a few ways to be with and honor this part of the self.

Full Moon Elemental Ritual Bath

This self-nurturing ritual blends the powers of the full moon and the four elements including select herbs, some suitable options being chamomile, lavender, tulsi, motherwort, and jasmine. The idea here is to take time to slow down and mindfully experience your own sensuality. Instead of overhead lighting, opt for atmospheric candlelight. Add a handful of herbs (or the tea from them) to a bath. Here, among the water, fire of the candles, herbs, and full moon, you are able to simply be—without the judgment of others and most importantly, without judgment from yourself. Allow yourself to be comforted and to find pleasure in the scent of the herbs, the feel of the warm water on your skin, the sound of water with each movement of your body, and the sight of the candle flames illuminating your surroundings. Focus on your breathing and how it feels as the air enters and leaves your lungs. Be mindful that you are an imperfectly perfect manifestation of Earth, Air, Fire, Water, and Spirit—a beloved child of Earth, the Great Mother.

Mothering the Inner Child

We all come into adulthood with past hurts and traumas tucked away into the depths of our psyches where we hope to keep them hidden. The problem is, even when we're avoiding past hurts, they're still there hiding in plain sight, and they're affecting how we operate and behave in daily life whether we realize it or not. As children, when we experience pain, we inevitably develop defense mechanisms to prevent such pain in the future. For example, if loud playing and raucous laughter infuriates a caregiver and results in physical punishment, the child will most likely become self-conscious and introverted in order to prevent similar reactions from the caregiver in the future. These defense mechanisms are then carried into adulthood where they no longer serve the same purpose, but they're now part of the brain's hardwiring. Because I witnessed violence against women during my childhood, I developed an aggressive protectiveness over others, particularly women, as well as myself. Inevitably, my learned defense mechanism followed me into adulthood resulting in problematic situations, and I had to reevaluate my innate response patterns. One way I've dealt with this is by approaching the child version of myself in my mind and comforting her (me) as she witnesses the violence that resulted in such behaviors. I explain to her that it is not her responsibility to protect adults from other adults, and that she is not a failure for not being able to do so. I tell her how proud of her I am that she feels the need to protect others from bullies and that in the future she will be able to channel these protective urges in more positive, productive ways. Try reaching out to the child version of yourself and comforting them as they experience a painful situation that has stuck with you after all these years. Be the source of stability and love that your younger self needed in those moments.

Mothering the Present Self

The love and comfort that a mother or caregiver provides is not just relevant to a child. While some might refuse to admit such vulnerability, we need the same kind of care in adulthood, but in a modified way. Just as you made yourself available to the hurt child in you, do the very same for the *you* that's right here, right now. Chances are your life isn't perfect and comes with its own brand of difficulties and stresses. Maybe you struggle with self-esteem issues and, as a result, tend to think and wrongly believe harsh thoughts about yourself. Maybe you tell yourself that you're stupid or ugly or not good enough. Now think back to the child version of you—I'm guessing you would never say the same harsh things to that child, but rather, you'd want to lift them up and encourage self-confidence. Afford your present self the same compassion because, whether you believe it or not, you deserve it as much as anyone. Hail, Berkana!

CORRESPONDENCES OF BERKANA

ELEMENT	Earth
ZODIAC	Cancer
PLANET	Moon
MOON PHASE	All
TAROT	The Empress, Queen of Swords
CRYSTAL	Chrysocolla
CHAKRA	Heart
DEITIES	Berchta, Demeter, Erzulie, Frigga, Gaia, Isis, Pachamama
PLANTS	Birch, Chamomile, Dong Quai, Flax, Motherwort, Rose of Jericho, Shatavari, Tulsi

The plants of Berkana embody femininity and motherhood. They are sensual, creative, and nurturing. The following plants are perfect for magick regarding fertility, pregnancy, and the birthing process as well as the protection of children and those in labor.

Birch
(*Betula* spp.)

The birch tree, also called "lady of the woods," is Berkana manifest. Birch trees represent the Divine Feminine and are especially sacred to the goddesses Freyja and Aino. Some say the wood of a birch should not be used unless the tree has been blessed by Thor (struck by lightning). Lore states that causing harm to the tree will anger the spirits of the forest. Because the birch offers the protection of a loving mother, fallen twigs are brought into the home to protect against curses and evil spirits. The lady of the woods represents love, new beginnings, protection, feminine magick, and the cycles of life and death. The wood is an excellent choice for rune and wand making; just be sure to first ask permission of the Great Goddess or the tree itself. When giving worship to the Earth Mother or the land spirits, offerings are best placed at the base of a birch tree.

Medicinal Properties

Tea prepared from birch leaves promotes healthy kidney and liver function, soothes coughs, and relieves indigestion. The bark targets urinary tract infections while the sap is cleansing to the blood. A decoction of the leaves helps to dissolve kidney stones. Birch essential oil offers relief for eczema, psoriasis, sore muscles, and arthritis. Actions: alterative, antibacterial, anti-inflammatory, antiseptic, astringent, cholagogue, diaphoretic, digestive, diuretic, nutritive, stimulant. Warming and drying. Avoid during pregnancy and nursing. Those who are easily dehydrated or with high blood pressure should avoid ingesting birch. Birch remedies should only be used under the supervision of a healthcare professional.

Chamomile
(*Matricaria recutita*)

Initially I had chamomile with Fehu due to its association with luck, success, and fortune. However, I've always gotten more of a motherly vibe from her. Such feelings preceded the realization that the genus name *Matricaria* comes from the Latin *mater* meaning "mother."

Chamomile is a nurturer that seeks to comfort those with emotional, mental, or physical sensitivities. You'll often find it in "calming" and "sleepy time" tea blends. It is a wonderful ally for healing trauma, comforting one's inner child, and moving out stagnant emotions. Call on the nurturing strength of Berkana while sipping warm chamomile tea when you feel the need for motherly love. Chamomile is one of the few herbs ruled by both the moon *and* the sun, so it makes sense that she's not only motherly but she's also lady luck! After all, mothers are far more than just that. In magick it can be tempting to compartmentalize correspondences into neat little boxes, but that would only limit our experiences with them. Chamomile is an herb of good luck. Traditionally, it has been grown in gardens to keep bad luck at bay. It promotes successful endeavors of any kind. Taking a trip to the casino? Wash your hands in the tea and draw Fehu in the center of your palm before hitting the tables. On the flip side, this gentle herb works well for promoting healthy money habits and discouraging greed. This is where we see those sun and moon energies blending. It can help one remember to focus on what they have rather than what they do not have.

Medicinal Properties

Chamomile is quite popular and is often added to tea blends for its deeply relaxing effects. Nothing beats a hot cup of chamomile at the end of a hectic day or times when emotions are running high. It has an affinity for the stomach, especially when stomach upset is the result of emotional distress. It is safe for children and helps to relieve hyperactivity, irritability, colds, and flu. As a topical, it soothes a multitude of skin conditions such as dermatitis, burns, acne, and eczema among others. Use as a gargle for sore throats and tooth pain. Actions: mild analgesic, antibacterial, antifungal, antihistamine, anti-inflammatory, antispasmodic, aromatic, carminative, diaphoretic, digestive, emetic, febrifuge, nervine, sedative, vulnerary. Neutral and moistening. Avoid essential oil during pregnancy. Avoid alongside anticoagulants. Large doses may cause vomiting.

Dong Quai
(*Angelica sinensis*)

Dong quai is protective and sacred to women. It promotes courage and confidence in women, especially during major transitions such as maiden to mother and from mother to crone. These titles more so denote the stages of one's life rather than whether one is a parent. Its soothing nature helps diffuse anger when there are disagreements in the home. Place near, but out of reach of, a baby to keep them safe while they sleep. Call on dong quai and Berkana to watch over and protect mother and baby during childbirth. Drink an infusion when performing rituals to reclaim personal sovereignty and/or sexuality. Dong quai is an ideal offering for any goddess and one I often gift to Lilith.

Medicinal Properties

Dong quai is a treasured tonic for women used widely within traditional Chinese medicine. It balances hormones such as estrogen and progesterone, which in turn encourages a healthy libido, regulates menstruation, and eases the pain of menstrual cramping. Dong quai promotes circulation and rebuilds blood after loss via menstruation and childbirth. Actions: alterative, anticoagulant, anti-inflammatory, antispasmodic, emmenagogue, estrogenic, nutritive, tonic. Warming and moistening. Avoid during pregnancy, nursing, and during extremely heavy periods. Dong quai exacerbates diarrhea.

Flax
(*Linum usitatissimum*)

Frigga, wife of Odin and queen of the Aesir, is often depicted holding her distaff, spinning flax into golden threads, or weaving the clouds in the sky. She is the goddess of motherhood and holds the ability to see into the future. Like Frigga, flax is protective of children and pregnancies and ideal for fertility workings. Fine linen fabrics, made from the fibrous seeds, were often the material used for ritual cloths and robes. The oil, called linseed oil, is used for the consecration of divination tools. Powdered incense made from the dried flowers promotes grounding, protection, and focus.

Medicinal Properties

Flax seed, also known as linseed, effectively targets inflammation of the gut. The high fiber content counters frequent constipation. Flax helps soothe chronic coughs, emphysema, bronchitis, and sore throat. It is balancing to hormones during menopause. The oil relieves common skin problems such as boils, lacerations, and rashes. The seeds should be ground up before swallowing. Be sure to stay hydrated when consuming flax seeds. Actions: anticancer, demulcent, emollient, estrogenic, laxative, nutritive. Cooling and moistening.

Motherwort
(*Leonurus cardiaca*)

Motherwort is truly a lion-hearted herb and one for those who could use a bit of encouraging and nurturing. It seeks to comfort, particularly those in the process of healing emotional wounds. As a guardian of women and plant of fertility magick, motherwort offers loving protection during pregnancy and childbirth. Hang a bundle in the home to promote joy and maternal protection while discouraging unwanted spirits from entering. Keep some with you to encourage strength and banish depression. Drink an infusion to promote self-love and an overall sense of peace. Motherwort is a wonderful offering for maternal deities such as Frigga, Isis, Demeter, and Gaia.

Medicinal Properties

Motherwort is supportive of cardiac health, remedying angina, arrhythmia, palpitations, and rapid heartbeat while strengthening overall heart function. It dulls the pains of childbirth and helps prevent postbirth infection. Take in tincture form to regulate the menstrual cycle and relieve cramps. As a bitter, motherwort has an affinity for the digestive system and supports healthy liver function. Its cardiac-nervine properties ease stress, anxiety, and nervousness and promote relaxation without drowsiness. For those who are recovering from illness, this herb will help to mother them back to health. Actions: antifungal, antispasmodic, antiviral, anxiolytic, astringent, bitter, cardiotonic, diaphoretic, emmenagogue, nervine, sedative, vasodilator. Cooling and drying.

While it should be avoided over the course of pregnancy, it may be used at the very end. Avoid during heavy periods.

Rose of Jericho
(*Selaginella lepidophylla*)

Rose of Jericho, also known as resurrection plant, is an ancient plant known for its ability to "come back to life" after appearing to dry out and die. This desert plant can go without water for up to a couple of years and will become resuscitated when watered. Such qualities fit in seamlessly with Berkana's powers of rebirth. Call on the Rose of Jericho to protect and fortify the spirit or when personal rebirth seems inevitable. Rose of Jericho is ideal for love magick, particularly with the reigniting of an old flame. It may be used to effectively remove the evil eye. In religious rites, Rose of Jericho water may be used in place of holy water. In Mexico, it was often placed in water at the onset of labor to foretell if delivery would be easy or complicated.

Medicinal Uses

There's very little information available on the medicinal properties of Rose of Jericho. What we do know of this Mexican native is that it has been used to treat infertility in women, menstrual cramping, labor pains, and to facilitate childbirth. The hot tea is soothing for sore throat and cold. Actions: antioxidant, diuretic, emmenagogue, vulnerary.

Shatavari
(*Asparagus racemosus*)

Shatavari embodies *Shakti*—a Hindu term describing the dynamic feminine aspect of divine energy. It exudes the sensuality and beauty of female sexuality. The name *shatavari* itself literally means "one hundred spouses" and most likely received its name due to its ability to enhance the libido and increase the chances of conception. Shatavari is perfect for sex, love, and fertility magick. It's ideal for rituals of feminine empowerment, sexual empowerment, and as offerings to deities like Parvati, Lilith, Oshun, and Freyja to name a few. It is an ally for those who have been sexually harmed by another, offering its energies to the healing of such traumas and rebuilding of confidence. While performing fertility magick, draw the Berkana rune over the womb with a mixture of oil and powdered shatavari.

Medicinal Properties

Shatavari is a potent rejuvenative. Like any adaptogen, it has myriad remedial uses, some of which include prevention of miscarriage, treating gastric ulcers, easing menopause, treating dehydration, and increasing breastmilk production. Overall, it is strengthening to those with weak and tired conditions, such as anemia or chronic fatigue. It possesses antiaging qualities and the ability to improve the memory. Shatavari is cleansing to the blood, treats uterine disorders, and counters impotence. It may be infused with oils or ghee to create a topical that promotes strong healthy skin. Actions: adaptogen, alterative, antibacterial, anti-inflammatory, anticancer, antioxidant, antispasmodic, aphrodisiac, demulcent, digestive, diuretic, galactagogue, immunostimulant, neuroprotective, nutritive. Cold and moistening.

Tulsi
(*Ocimum sanctum*)

To get an idea of tulsi's energies, one must only learn some of the plant's other names, which are holy basil or *Bhutagni,* meaning "destroyer of demons." Sacred in India, it is an herb of nurturing and harmony and is especially balancing to the chakra system. Tulsi is a motherly herb that seeks to protect spiritually, mentally, and physically. It is evocative of Lakshmi, the Hindu goddess of love, joy, and health, and also of Vishnu, one of the supreme creators of the universe along with Shiva and Brahma. Like Lakshmi, tulsi is loving, joyful, and serene but also strongly capable of repelling harmful energy. It strengthens the qualities of compassion and generosity. Tulsi is traditionally employed magickally for purification and exorcism. It is stabilizing to the mind and helps to clear away psychic pollution. To attract new love, hang a bundle outside the front door or bedroom window. A leaf placed in the mouth of the dying ensures a peaceful transition from this life to the next.

Medicinal Properties

Tulsi improves vitality and works to heal the damage caused by stress. It works to lower blood pressure and cholesterol, stabilize blood sugar, and relieve respiratory complaints such as hay fever, cough, and asthma. It's been used to lower fevers, improve cognitive function, relieve diarrhea, and even repel mosquitos. It encourages appetite and eases gastrointestinal upsets in children. As a topical, tulsi remedies both bacterial and fungal infections of the skin. Many adaptogens benefit pets just as they benefit humans; every morning I sprinkle a couple of pinches of powdered tulsi on my dogs' food as a supplemental boost. Actions: adaptogen, analgesic, antibacterial, anticancer, antidepressant, anti-inflammatory, antioxidant, antispasmodic, antiviral, anxiolytic, carminative, diaphoretic, digestive, diuretic, expectorant, febrifuge, galactagogue, heart tonic, immunostimulant, nootropic, stomachic. Cooling and drying.

19

EHWAZ

ᛖ

Phonetic equivalent: E
Horse, Trust, Relationships

Ehwaz hands to me the reins
Upon the horse I ride
A trusted ally as I journey
A source of love and pride

Ehwaz (pronounced eh-wahz) translates to "horse," a sacred animal in ancient Germanic culture, and represents the symbiotic relationship that has long been held by humans and horses. Horses have long been used as a method of transportation; thus, the rune illustrates the importance of trust and loyalty between the animal and rider. In return for the horse's sacrifice, the human must tend to the needs of the animal. Additional meanings of Ehwaz are movement, cooperation, changing directions, anima, subjectivity, emotion, love, and animals. If Raidho is the rune of travel, Ehwaz represents the vehicle in which to travel. Modern correspondences include cars, trains, bikes, and the like.

Not only did horses provide a means of transportation but they also provided companionship. The animals we welcome into our lives, whether for service or general companionship, very often become family. The friendship between human and animal can be just as profound as exclusively human friendships. From this we are able to make sense of the Ehwaz rune's meaning as both the horse rune and the love/emotion rune. Ehwaz covers all categories of love, including romantic love, and is considered the wedding or union rune. Symbolically, it is used to strengthen love, promote fidelity, and bestow good luck upon a romantic relationship.

In matters of psychology, Ehwaz represents the ability to adjust and adapt to the inevitable changes in life. Do we accept or resist? Do we move with or against the current? Life, like a horse, can change direction swiftly. The "rider" must be prepared for anything, or they risk falling off, literally and metaphorically.

Ehwaz is associated with Carl Jung's concept of the anima. The anima is the feminine energy contained within everyone, and its opposite, the animus, is the masculine energy in all. Anima refers to breath, vital force, spirit, subjectivity, emotion, and the inward flow of energy. Animus is mind, rationale, objectivity, desire, and the outward flow of energy. On one end of the spectrum is anima, and on the other is animus, and every single being in the cosmos falls somewhere in between. When gender is considered in terms of spectrums and ratios, we are able to better understand gender fluidity. Today more than ever, we understand how the concept of binary genders is oversimplified. We all float somewhere on the spectrum, and it's a long way from point A to point B.

In readings Ehwaz typically refers to partnerships, the momentum of a situation, what direction one should take, emotional health, and love. If it shows up in a reading with Raidho, it may indicate a literal journey in the near future. Alongside Gebo, Ehwaz can illustrate the importance of balanced give and take within a relationship. Murkstave Ehwaz may indicate ending a relationship, mistrust, enemies, betrayal, frustration, mismanaged emotions, disputes, and a lack of momentum or stagnation.

Ehwaz helps us better connect to nature through our friends in the animal kingdom, and one doesn't have to have animals in their home to do so. Whether we have in-the-flesh familiars, family pets, or spirit animals who reside in other realms, there is much to learn from our companions.

While mostly shielded from the wild, domesticated animals still display behaviors that only served them well in nature. Dogs bury their bones (my dog Lunar tries to bury his bone in his bed, and it's adorable) and cats bring home their daily catches as gifts—a habit that stems from wild cats bringing meals home to feed their young. My cat Sabbath loves to catch mice and bring them home for me. Thanks, I think? I highlight these behaviors because no matter how domesticated, you just can't take the wild out of the animal; and that goes for humans as well. We are all, at our foundations, wild animals—a notion that brings with it a sense of real freedom.

One way to work with animals in magick is through bones and other remains. Many are against this, and I understand why. I only collect bones that have been found outdoors. Hunting and killing animals for the purpose of acquiring bones and/or pelts is something I am vehemently against.

Bones and other remains carry with them fragments of the spirit that once inhabited them. Whenever I come across bones on hikes, I make sure to sit with them for a moment to get a sense of whether they're content with being an ally of mine. A few times I have come across bones or remains that gave off strong "leave me be!" vibes. The ones that don't mind coming home with me are cleaned, consecrated, and rehomed on one of my altars. Once a relationship is established, I present the bones with offerings in exchange for aid in my magickal workings. Coyote bones offer fast and sly energies, bird wings may be used to represent the element of Air, and badger bones are fitting for hexing and banishing. Some of the bones that I have are a mystery to me, and I tend to use those specifically for their death energy during dark moon rituals or as a symbol for endings.

When participating in otherworldly travel, having a spirit animal (also known as a totem) is invaluable. Some spirit animals are stalwart protectors while others impart valuable wisdom and magickal knowledge. Some are easygoing while others are more inclined to show tough love. Some are temporary, while others are lifelong. Part of the process of taking on a spirit animal companion is trusting that we are given who we need when we need them. Intuition is of immense importance when we are putting our trust in otherworldly beings. Not every entity that presents itself to us has harmless intentions; one of the great benefits of traveling with a companion is that extra sense of discernment.

However you choose to work with animals in your practice, the most important thing is to show them the respect they deserve. They have much to teach us. The ones that we welcome into our homes and families bring us amazing gifts of unconditional love—it's no wonder animals are represented by the rune of love.

An important lesson we can learn from animals is how to be accepting and mindful. They very much live in the here and now. They seem largely unburdened by a need to define themselves or present themselves in any way other than exactly who they are. Observe the animals around you, the ones in your home or the wild animals outside of your home. They do not care that we are *pagans, witches,* or *humans* . . . titles and labels mean nothing to them. Challenge the very way in which you view yourself. Who are you beneath the titles, labels, and expectations of society? When and how often does the wild animal inside of you come out? If you haven't, try the applicable Onion Ritual on page 164. If you have animals at home, consider who you are in their eyes; and just like them, choose to live in your truth always. Hail, Ehwaz!

CORRESPONDENCES OF EHWAZ

ELEMENT	Water
ZODIAC	Pisces
PLANET	Neptune
MOON PHASE	Waxing
TAROT	2 of Cups
CRYSTAL	Rhodochrosite
CHAKRA	Sacral
DEITIES	Áine, Artemis, Epona, Karærin, Parvati, Rhiannon
PLANTS	Cleavers, Linden, Lovage, Marjoram, Milky Oat, Red Clover, Rose, Skullcap

The following plants of Ehwaz are of a gentle nature, ideal for workings in love, trust, and healing. They are especially protective of animals and work to strengthen the bonds between humans and the rest of the animal kingdom.

Cleavers
(*Gallium aparine*)

Because cleavers are sticky and tend to grab on to anything they come in contact with, they are often used to help the practitioner obtain that which is desired. Cleavers symbolize manifestation, making it a popular plant for love and money spells. Add them to incense blends or hang bundles at weddings to attract luck and strength to the union. To make a charm for the blessing of a union, use twigs and twine to construct an Ehwaz rune and finish it by wrapping fresh cleavers around the twigs. Hang over the couple's shared bed, or if a wedding is underway, place it above the altar where the couple will exchange vows.

Medicinal Properties
Cleavers help to cleanse the blood and detoxify the lymphatic system and kidneys. They tone, tighten, and improve skin while treating acne, eczema, psoriasis, neurofibromatosis, abscesses, sunburn, and bug bites. Apply as a poultice for wound care. The strong diuretic aspects of cleavers are unrivaled for treating urinary tract infections and bladder infections and dissolving kidney stones. They work to lower high blood pressure. The roots of the plant are effective in relieving stubborn toothaches. Actions: alterative, anticancer, anti-inflammatory, astringent, diaphoretic, diuretic, febrifuge, hepatic, kidney tonic, vulnerary. Cooling and drying. Avoid alongside diabetes.

Linden
(*Tilia* spp.)

Is it a coincidence that the linden tree sports heart-shaped leaves while at the same time relating energetically to love and healthy emotion? The doctrine of signatures tells us it is not. Linden lends its magickal abilities to the strengthening of love by promoting relationship health and longevity. This is not only ideal for romance but for friend and family relationships as well. The energies of linden are calming and comforting and help to soothe the frazzled mind, which is necessary before performing any kind of magick. The flowers in particular are heart-healing and motivational, and they work to imbue those nearby with hope and optimism. In German lore, the linden tree was considered a home for magickal creatures such as dragons, faeries, and elves.

Medicinal Properties

Linden, also known as lime tree, is a valued medicine thanks to its ability to target and fight cold and flu symptoms such as sinus congestion and pain, sore throat, cough, and fever. It encourages the release of serotonin, a neurotransmitter that is necessary for mood stability. The flowers are emollient, which supports smooth, healthy skin by strengthening elasticity. Linden tea is a quick and easy way to treat inflammatory conditions such as tension, arthritis, headaches, and gout. Actions: anti-inflammatory, antispasmodic, anxiolytic, decongestant, diaphoretic, emollient, sedative. Cooling and drying. Avoid excessive use alongside heart disease. Avoid if pregnant or nursing.

Lovage
(*Levisticum officinale*)

Lovage isn't just a plant of love, it's a plant of *self*-love. It reminds one to be gentle with oneself and encourages self-prioritization. Lovage is a plant ally for those who tend to suffer from low confidence. It can, of course, also be applied to love that involves others. If you're hoping to meet someone new, add a lovage leaf and a bindrune of Ehwaz and Kenaz to a sachet or charm and keep it on your person. If possible, renew the leaf once every couple of days until you succeed in meeting that special someone—and don't forget to put yourself out there. Performing magick to attract a new partner is useless if you aren't actively meeting new people.

Medicinal Properties

Lovage is ideal for urinary health. It is an aquaretic, which means it encourages increased urination without the loss of electrolytes. It also helps to prevent kidney stones. Lovage may be used to treat both dys-menorrhea and amenorrhea. Additionally, this perennial benefits indigestion, poor circulation, and bronchitis. It reduces irritation of the lungs and dissolves phlegm of the respiratory tract. Poultices or salves made from the root benefit skin disorders and joint pain. The ripened seeds may be chewed to aid in proper digestion. Actions: antibacterial, aquaretic, carminative, diaphoretic, digestive, diuretic, emmenagogue, expectorant, stimulant. Warm and drying. Avoid during pregnancy and nursing. Avoid alongside kidney disease.

Marjoram
(*Origanum majorana*)

Marjoram is a magickal herb of purification, love, and protection. Its energies target and heal strained relationships. It helps in matters of finding a prospective partner while protecting against those who harbor ill intentions. As an herb of love, marjoram is sacred to the Aphrodite, Greek goddess of love and beauty. An offering of marjoram is perfect for any deity befitting the lover archetype including Parvati, Venus, Hathor, and Freyja. It does not work well for lust and simple attractions but rather when true companionship and lasting love is desired. Marjoram is also a funereal herb and suitable for death, burial rites, and to help with the grief of those left behind. Being an herb of love, beauty, and death, it's the perfect offering at the graves of loved ones, especially during Samhain. If marjoram is not available, oregano is a suitable replacement.

Medicinal Properties

Marjoram is soothing for headaches, toothaches, excessive flatulence, indigestion, edema, and respiratory complaints. It is beneficial for those who suffer from insomnia or anxiety. The essential oil is used as a stress reliever and mood booster. Add the herb or a few drops of the essential oil to a nighttime bath to promote relaxation of the mind and body. Traditionally, the powdered herb has been used as a snuff to induce sneezing. Marjoram is high in antioxidants and protects the skin against the harmful effects of free radicals. Actions: antibacterial, antifungal, antispasmodic, carminative, diaphoretic, digestive, diuretic, emmenagogue, expectorant, nervine, stimulant. Warming and drying. Avoid essential oil during pregnancy.

Milky Oats
(*Avena sativa*)

If plants could give hugs, milky oat would be the first to wrap its stems around you when comfort is needed. It is associated with the new moon and new beginnings and supports the reinvention of self, especially after periods of difficulty. Milky oats benefit those recovering from substance addiction and help to provide some of the support necessary in early sobriety. Increase and prosperity also fall under the expertise of this encouraging plant, making it a fitting option for ingredients in abundance charms and potions. In Scotland, oat cakes called bannocks are a traditional treat for sabbat celebrations.

Medicinal Properties

Milky oats are simply oats before they are fully ripened. They make a wonderful plant remedy for children who are hyperactive, ADHD, or easily agitated. The oats may be given as a tea or added to bathwater. Oat baths are a fantastic way to soothe itchy skin, eczema, neuralgia, and fibromyalgia. The high silicon content works to strengthen hair, skin, and nails. Because it is helpful in balancing and strengthening the nervous system, milky oat works well for those recovering from substance addiction. It helps to relieve tension headaches, PMS, post-traumatic stress response, depression, nervous exhaustion, and imbalanced hormones. Milky oat treats convalescence and debility while increasing stamina. Historically, it was used as a medicine for leprosy. Actions: antidepressant, alterative, demulcent, diaphoretic, diuretic, emollient, nervine, nutritive, tonic. Neutral and moistening. Use caution alongside gluten allergies.

Red Clover
(*Trifolium pratense*)

Red clover brings luck and purity to any magick it's applied to and is particularly useful in matters of love, protection, cleansing, and money.

It has a fondness for domestic animals and seeks to protect them from illness and predators. Red clover also provides comfort for those facing the loss of a beloved animal. I have an altar dedicated to my animals that have passed, where I keep their ashes, jars of fur, paw-prints, photos, and plenty of red clover. Bathe in the blossoms or add to a decorative bouquet to attract prosperity and love. If the elusive four-leaf clover is spotted, add it to a luck charm and keep it with you to attract good fortune.

Medicinal Properties

The gorgeous puffy blossoms of red clover make a pleasantly sweet herbal tea that supports overall health and wellness. Red clover deeply cleanses blood, strengthens bones, supports heart health, and balances hormones. It effectively treats various skin conditions like burns, psoriasis, and eczema and even provides topical soothing for skin cancer. It is a suitable remedy for respiratory ailments that result in severe coughs. Red clover contains phytoestrogens, which support the relief of menopause symptoms, hot flashes in particular. It may prevent estrogen-dependent cancers and has been used in holistic treatments for breast cancer sufferers. Red clover may be taken to alleviate cramps and sore breasts during menstruation. Actions: alterative, analgesic, antispasmodic, cholagogue, diaphoretic, diuretic, estrogenic, expectorant, lymphatic, nervine, nutritive, pectoral, vulnerary. Cooling and balancing.

Rose
(*Rosa* spp.)

Also known as the "queen of flowers," the rose is the epitome of love and beauty. The energies of this Venusian flower are perfect for love spells of any kind. In my personal experience with roses, I have learned how powerful they are for helping one care for and love themselves. The flowers or petals may be offered during invocations of the Divine Feminine, as well as to ancestors and deities. Include petals in aphrodisiac elixirs, teas, and incense. As a symbol of femininity, it has a strong connection to lunar magick. Roses of any color are a popular choice for wedding bouquets and decor to create an atmosphere of love. The parts of this well-known flower can be used for various types of magick. In chapter 1, we spoke of rose hips' affinity for success. The thorns are symbolic of Thurisaz and work well in defensive magick. And let's not forget about color magick—red for romance, pink for friendship, yellow for joy, and white for innocence and spirituality. Add the petals to baths before an evening of *l'amour* or simply when you want to treat yourself to a bit of luxury. With a spoon, trace an Ehwaz rune in rose tea to counter feelings of cynicism and apathy. As you sip the tea, take in feelings of gratitude and love.

Medicinal Properties

Rose possesses a cooling effect that soothes burns and quells "hot" anger. Rosewater sprays are a simple and effective remedy for sunburns. The astringency treats excessive mucus, hemorrhoids, and diarrhea. The essential oil is used in aromatherapy to relax and ease melancholic states. Rose helps to lower high cholesterol. Actions: alterative, antibacterial, antidepressant, antioxidant, antispasmodic, aphrodisiac, astringent, cardiotonic, decongestant, expectorant, refrigerant, sedative. Cooling and drying.

Skullcap
(*Scutellaria lateriflora*)

Skullcap is binding to oaths, contracts, and vows and is therefore a perfect herb for initiations and weddings. It ensures fidelity within romantic relationships. For relationships in need of repair or steeped in anger, skullcap helps to soften hard emotions and replace resentment with compassion. Use in spells to bring about reconciliation among friends, lovers, or family members. For those who live with their romantic partner(s), keep a bit of skullcap and an Ehwaz rune under the mattress of the bed to ensure faithfulness and a blessed union. Replace every couple of months to keep the energies fresh. Skullcap is an incredible herb to use in spells and rituals for removing addiction. It works well to anchor one's spirit to the body during trance and astral travel. Because of its nervine and sedative qualities, skullcap is quite beneficial for entering deep meditation and trance.

Medicinal Properties

Skullcap is tranquil and relaxing, helping to soothe upsets like insomnia, ADHD, fear, and a generally chaotic mind. It treats nervous stomach and the indigestion that tends to accompany it. Skullcap is an ideal remedy for colds, tension headaches, and dizziness. It increases endorphins, which help to relieve the shock of drug or alcohol withdrawal for those in the process of substance detox. Actions: analgesic, antibacterial, antioxidant, antispasmodic, anxiolytic, astringent, bitter, diuretic, hypotensive, neuroprotective, nervine, sedative, spinal cord tonic, vasodilator. Cold and drying. Use sparingly as overuse may cause damage to the liver. Avoid during pregnancy and nursing.

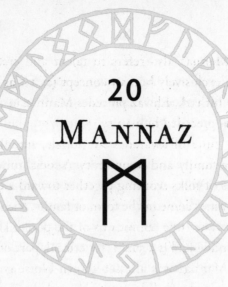

20
MANNAZ

Phonetic equivalent: M
Humanity, Community, Intelligence

Mannaz is humanity
Awareness, conscious mind
Our tribes provide support
Never a member left behind

Mannaz (pronounced man-ahz) translates to "mankind" or "human"—an easy one to remember given the name. In chapter 19 we discussed animals, anima, emotion, and subjectivity. With Mannaz we will focus on humanity, animus, logic, and objectivity. These runes are two sides of the same coin and together promote balance.

While Ehwaz and Mannaz are similar in appearance, what separates the two is Gebo—the rune of gifts, reciprocity, and harmony—which is found in the Mannaz rune. The shape of the rune also calls to mind an image of two people facing one another in an embrace. Humans need other humans for many reasons, and people who are part of collectives need to be able to rely on one another. Without mutual support and proper give and take, the structure of a relationship or community is weakened and can potentially fall apart. Humans are innately community-driven, seeking like-minded individuals for friendships and partnerships. Mannaz also refers to talent and creativity, which implies the arts, an exclusively human concept (as far as we know). In the sequence of the futhark, Ehwaz precedes Mannaz just as the rest of the animal kingdom preceded humanity.

Mannaz is the rune of awareness, rationale, intelligence, talent, analysis, social order, family, and community. A social rune, it represents united communities of folks working together toward a common goal. Today such communities come in the form of family, friends, coworkers, coven, or neighbors. The rune reminds us of the potential of the collective and how each individual is a small, yet crucial, part of a whole.

In mythology, Mannaz was a lesser-known Norse god, said to the be the forefather from which all humans descended. The rune also has connections with the watchman of the gods, Heimdall, who resides on the bridge between Midgard and Asgard.

Psychologically, Mannaz is the rune of academia. It is known as a *hugrune,* a rune of mind and thought. This term comes from Odin's ravens, Huginn (thought) and Muninn (memory). Mannaz refers to objectivity and logic. It is the animus within us all, regardless of gender or lack thereof.

In readings, Mannaz may be asking one to analyze their part in a community or group. It may indicate the need to ask for or offer help. If it appears alongside Ansuz, the reading might indicate the importance of healthy communication. With Othala, it is likely that one's immediate family is being called to attention. Additional meanings include thought patterns, study, and the need for structure. Murkstave, the humanity rune can indicate misanthropy, ostracism, isolation, selfishness, illogical or irrational thoughts, or enemies.

When I was considering the ways in which Mannaz contributes to the rewilding process, it occurred to me that the hugrune can be helpful in illustrating what can be detrimental to the human-nature connection, and that is a mindset based solely on logic. That is not to say logic is second to abstract, intuitive thought, because that's just not true. Both are of immense importance in this thing we call life. They balance each other out. Certain situations, however, may call for more of one over the other.

Like magick and witchcraft, nature cannot be approached with only logic and intellect—feeling and heart are equally, if not more, essential. As an example, I'll briefly touch on my first couple of years practicing trance meditation. In a nutshell, they were extremely frustrating. No matter how much I read and learned about the subject, I just could not successfully enter a trance state. I tried every technique I could find, but time and time again I was met with disappointment. Eventually I realized that I was approaching the practice of trance from an exclusively intellectual point of view. Here's the thing about trance—you can't *think* yourself into it. When I stopped trying to "figure out" and just "let go," I was able to find success in achieving trance. Easier said than done, of course, but I eventually got it. The same sentiment can apply to magick and communing with nature. In order to successfully do these things, we have to let go of traditional methods of thought and activate a subtler part of ourselves. There's an element of surrender that is necessary for these things.

In chapter 4 we discussed communication with the world around us—specifically, with plants. In it I discussed my previous struggle with such communication and how I experienced the same kind of disappointment and realization regarding my solely logical approach. I'm a Capricorn sun and a Virgo moon—I'm plagued with an overly analytical mind. Skepticism and overthinking are my superpowers. When I resumed my witchcraft practice in adulthood I had to consciously make a point to suspend disbelief. I actually wrote "suspend disbelief" in every box of my datebook for months as a reminder. Thankfully over time I've gotten much better at doing so.

Interestingly, scientists believe that intuitive thought happens near the pineal gland, which is often referred to as the third eye. The appearance of the pineal gland is often compared to the Eye of Horus. Spiritualists consider this part of the brain to be the seat of the soul. The opening of the third eye begins with the exercising of intuition. This can be done via meditation, by becoming acquainted with dreams, or through various kinds of divination such as scrying, tarot, and runes.

The following meditation is meant to awaken the subtle, intuitive mind—think of it as a way to clear the sleep gunk out of the third eye. The more you practice this or similar types of meditation, the stronger your subtle senses will become.

Because the pineal gland is sensitive to vibration, begin the session with a singing bowl, bells, or soothing music in the background—something that you won't find distracting. Assume whatever meditation position works best for you. For me it is seated cross-legged on the floor with a pillow under my bum to keep my back from becoming achy. Before you start, you may choose to anoint the third eye with oil.

Close your eyes and rest your hands palms up. Take a few slow, deep breaths in through the nose and out through the mouth. With each in-breath imagine violet light pervading your torso, then spreading out to the arms, legs, and finally, throughout the head, where it stops and glows brightly at the pineal gland or third eye. Your whole body is now filled with violet light, but it is brightest at the third eye. Keep your attention there. Breathe normally. With each in-breath, "feel" and "see" the violet light becoming brighter and maybe even slightly pulsating along with the beat of your heart. Take notice of how the violet light feels. Is it warm? Tingly? Do you feel a bit light-headed? (Pun not intended.) Are any emotions coming up? Notice these things without analyzing or judgment.

Allow any random thoughts that pop up to gently pass by as if they're carried away in a stream. If you get distracted, simply return your attention to the third eye. Feel the eye open between your brows. Continue with the meditation until you feel it's complete. For folks who aren't used to meditation, increments of five to ten minutes are a great way to start. If the violet light has you feeling overly energized, place your feet and hands on the earth and allow the excess energy to flow into the ground. For best results, try this meditation during a full moon or during liminal times like the solstices and equinoxes. If possible, try it with a partner or a group. Afterall, Mannaz is all about community and the sharing of experiences. Share your impressions with one another.

Hail, Mannaz!

CORRESPONDENCES OF MANNAZ

ELEMENT	Air
ZODIAC	Virgo
PLANET	Mercury
MOON PHASE	Waxing
TAROT	The Emperor, Ace of Swords
CRYSTAL	Apatite
CHAKRA	Throat
DEITIES	Athena, Heimdall, Ogma, Papa Legba, Seshat, Tenjin, Thoth
PLANTS	Caraway, Ginkgo, Gotu Kola, Lemongrass, Rosemary, Spearmint

Caraway
(*Carum carvi*)

The seeds of caraway support those who seek to obtain true wisdom and keep an open mind. It strengthens memory, general cognitive function, and is an excellent study herb. Add them to dream pillows with mugwort and lavender to assist with dream recall. Lore states that any item containing caraway seeds cannot be stolen, and a wash made from the seeds may be used for the same purpose. Hanging bundles of the plant at the entrances of a home or business will deter thieves from entering, and placing a dish full of seeds beneath a child's crib will discourage any ill-intentioned entities from approaching.

Medicinal Properties

Caraway is quite similar in taste to anise and fennel and makes a delicious tea that effectively targets all types of indigestion. The seeds especially work to relieve heartburn, nausea, bloating, and excessive flatulence. Caraway seeds help to improve appetite, relieve coughs, ease menstrual cramping, and encourage the production of breastmilk. The seeds are a safe remedy for treating indigestion in children. Use as a gargle for sore throats. Actions: anticancer, antispasmodic, aromatic, carminative, digestive, diuretic, expectorant, galactagogue, stimulant, stomachic, tonic. Warming.

Ginkgo
(*Ginkgo biloba*)

After the nuclear bombing of Hiroshima, ginkgo was the first plant to regrow, and amazingly, it lacked genetic mutation. Six trees survived the blast and are alive and well today. Ginkgo represents resilience and is one of the oldest living plant species, going all the way back to the dinosaurs. In Japan the tree is regarded as sacred and is often planted at places of worship. This ancient tree of wisdom promotes intelligence, clarity, and inspiration. It is a true ally for those studying the occult arts and mysteries. As an elder of trees, ginkgo is ideal for longevity spells and communication with the ancestors. The seeds represent male fertility and lend their powers to various forms of love and reproductive magick. To stimulate the mind for divination, astral travel, or magick of any type, grind the dried leaves to a fine powder before adding to a bit of olive oil. Then use a finger to trace the Mannaz symbol on the forehead with the oil. Feel and imagine the symbol glowing a bright golden light and clearing away any mental fog that may hinder your work. This is also a great exercise for stimulating the memory.

Medicinal Properties

Perhaps best known for its ability to strengthen the memory and cognition, ginkgo leaf is a go-to for general brain health. It improves circulation to the brain, which in turn reduces the risk of stroke. It reduces the symptoms of dementia, anxiety, and some mental illnesses. Ginkgo helps relieve dizziness, tinnitus, altitude sickness, and vertigo. It's a powerful anti-inflammatory that works well in treating arthritis, irritable bowel syndrome, inflammation-related headaches, and multiple sclerosis. Ginkgo promotes eye health through improved circulation. It is used to treat male sexual dysfunction and is a valuable remedy for asthma and allergies. To relieve wheezing, ingest a decoction of the seeds. Actions: adaptogen, anticoagulant, anti-inflammatory, antioxidant, antispasmodic, anxiolytic, cerebral tonic, hypotensive, nootropic, vasodilator. Neutral. Avoid in excess as large doses may be toxic. Those who take anticoagulants should check with a healthcare professional before ingesting ginkgo.

Gotu Kola
(*Centella asiatica*)

Like ginkgo, gotu kola is a reinforcer of the mind. Because it's a plant of memory, burning it as incense is an appropriate offering to loved ones who have passed or ancestors in general, especially when paired with rosemary. Gotu kola may be applied to the development and balance of the crown chakra, enhancing psychic power along the way. It is ideal for countering forgetfulness and mental deterioration. Use alongside ginkgo and Mannaz to support peak mental function.

Medicinal Properties

Gotu kola is a brain food that supports healthy function, specifically concentration, alertness, and memory. It treats anxiety, amnesia, dementia, senility, and fatigue. As a rejuvenating longevity tonic, it is a wonderful supplement for the elderly. In ayurvedic medicine it is valued for its ability to repair tissue and is often applied topically to treat serious skin conditions such as leprosy. It also helps to prevent scarring. Gotu kola relieves arthritis pain and balances the adrenals. As a mild diuretic, it stimulates the release of excess toxins. Actions: adaptogen, anti-inflammatory, antioxidant, aphrodisiac, detoxifier, digestive, diuretic, nervine, nootropic, sedative, tonic, vulnerary. Cooling and drying. Those who take anticoagulants should check with a healthcare professional before ingesting gotu kola. Large doses may cause headache and dizziness. Avoid alongside overactive thyroid.

Lemongrass
(*Cymbopogon citratus*)

The energies of lemongrass possess a childlike innocence and purity—exactly the type of energies one would employ for mild cleansings. The incense provides a fresh lemon scent that encourages an open-minded outlook, enhanced memory, clear communication, mental clarity, creativity, and focus. Lemongrass aids the seeker in finding truth, especially regarding occult mysteries. As a tea or bathing herb, it helps prepare the practitioner for divination and other psychic tasks, while expelling heavy, unfavorable energies. Alongside its mind-strengthening qualities, lemongrass also has an affinity for love and attraction magick. Pair with Mannaz to facilitate success on a first date.

Medicinal Properties

Lemongrass soothes a variety of digestive complaints, such as flatulence and bloating. It is a mild yet effective digestive remedy for children. The essential oil stimulates mental alertness and helps ease mild depression. Massaged into the skin, the diluted oil relieves arthritis pain, muscle cramps and spasms, as well as fungal skin conditions like ringworm or athlete's foot. Lemongrass induces sweat, which helps to clear fevers. The hot tea brings relaxation to those who have trouble sleeping due to insomnia or anxiety. Lemongrass is a natural mosquito repellent. Actions: analgesic, antibacterial, anti-inflammatory, antiviral, anxiolytic, diaphoretic, digestive, sedative. Cooling.

Rosemary
(*Salvia rosmarinus*)

Rosemary is strongly associated with memory and concentration. It has ties to the god Odin, whose pair of ravens Huginn (thought) and Muninn (memory) fly around near and far collecting information for Odin. With its association to memory, rosemary is perfect for honoring and remembering loved ones who have passed on. It's an herb of Samhain due to its association with death and its protective qualities, which guard against the mischievous spirits that pass through the temporarily thinned veil. I typically employ rosemary for increasing focus and memory, especially during my studies. I'm a bookworm but I'm also easily distracted! If you're anything like me and tend to drift off and think about that embarrassing thing you did fifteen years ago, only to realize you've just read an entire page of a book, then rosemary is probably the herb for you! For individuals dealing with memory depletion, the pairing of Mannaz and rosemary strengthens cognitive function.

The heady smoke of rosemary incense is a strong purifier ideal for combatting illness and distress.

Medicinal Properties

Rosemary has been employed as a medicine in Africa, Asia, and Europe for almost ten thousand years. Today, it's still used to help improve memory and concentration. It boosts circulation to the brain and contains antioxidant properties that protect the blood vessels within. Because of its effects on the blood vessels of the brain, it may be helpful in treating headaches and migraines. Rosemary helps prevent and remedy memory depletion, depression, rheumatism, digestive upset, and low blood pressure. It is high in iron and vitamin C. It is a wonderful additive to topicals aimed at treating burns, wounds, eczema, psoriasis, and sciatica. Actions: antidepressant, antioxidant, antirheumatic, antiseptic, carminative, cerebral tonic, expectorant. Warming and drying. Rosemary is poisonous in large doses and should not be ingested long term. Avoid during pregnancy except in culinary amounts. Those with epilepsy should avoid the essential oil. Avoid alongside aspirin allergies.

Spearmint
(*Mentha spicata*)

The refreshing vibes of spearmint are perfect for purifying objects, spaces, and people. No matter how you choose to use it (e.g., tea, incense, essential oil) it promotes recovery, good health, renewal, and success. Like its close relative peppermint, spearmint is excellent for healing rituals, especially regarding ailments of the lungs. Use in any form to calm anger and anxiety. Spearmint encourages healthy communication between partners—whether lovers or business partners. Because it attracts peace and clarity of the mind, it's a true herbal ally for meditation. During times when you're feeling down or simply out of sorts, add to a bath to reset and uplift.

Medicinal Properties

Spearmint is milder than peppermint and is a wonderful herb for children's upsets such as hiccups, indigestion, vomiting, and fevers. Adding the essential oil to a diffuser can help relieve stress. For those who are pregnant and experiencing morning sickness (or afternoon or evening sickness), spearmint is a safe and mild remedy for the relieving of nausea. The taste and scent assist in deterring sugar cravings. Spearmint aids in the rebalancing of female hormones. When testosterone levels are high in women, it can result in unwanted facial hair; spearmint helps to combat this and lower the testosterone. Actions: analgesic, antioxidant, antispasmodic, antifungal, carminative, digestive, diuretic, febrifuge, stimulant, stomachic. Cooling, warming, and drying.

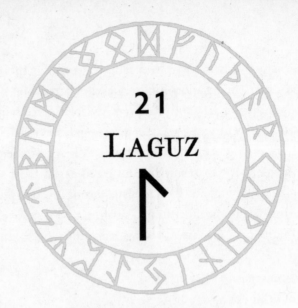

21
LAGUZ

Phonetic equivalent: L
Emotions, Intuition, Dreams

I am purified and blessed
As I swim within her depths
With the tide I ebb and flow
Where it takes me, I don't know

Laguz (pronounced lah-gooz) is one of four runes associated with the Divine Feminine, alongside Hagalaz, Perthro, and Berkana. It translates to *water* and possesses the classic occult characteristics of the Water element such as the lunar energy, intuition, emotion, dreams, psychic ability, and imagination. Laguz is arguably the patron rune of the völva (Norse female seer/witch) due to its association with subtle messages, spirit work, divination, and astral projection.

Because it's inextricably linked with magick and the moon, Laguz is a wonderful ally for magickal practitioners of any kind. It activates and encourages strengthening of the subtle senses so that we may better understand our environment and the energies within. It can help us as we explore our depths in search of our individual power.

It can help one sort through emotions that, like water, can manifest as a still pond or a raging tsunami. Water is life-giving, and we are beings of water ourselves—perhaps the main reason we are so affected by the phases of the moon. Like fire, water is both life-supporting and capable of immense harm. In turbulent waters we risk drowning. Metaphorically, this illustrates the importance of acknowledging our emotions and seeking support if they are unmanageable or the cause of suffering.

In a reading, Laguz may highlight one's current emotional state, love, depth, secrets, or intuition. If it shows up in a reading with Kenaz, the querant may be asked to shine a light on that which is being hidden below the surface. It asks one to pay attention to intuition and dreams. Paired with Mannaz it may indicate the need for emotional and logical balance. With Ansuz, it may be asking you to pay attention to the messages coming through in dreams. Reversed or murkstave it may point to blockage, unmanaged emotions, confusion, depression, nightmares, or spiritual neglect.

Laguz focuses on depth and the ability to see below the surface. It is a rune of complexity much like the human psyche. When Kenaz and Laguz are paired, the psychological implication is the surfacing of repressed memories. Like an iceberg, which is 90 percent below the water's surface, Laguz points out that we are rarely able to see a person or situation for exactly what it is. Humans are similar to icebergs in the way that our outward behaviors, which are often subjected to scrutiny from others, are products of an immensely large, yet not visible, conglomeration of experience below the surface. We are shaped by our experiences, good, neutral, and traumatic. The wisdom of Laguz teaches us that in order to better understand the surface we must first understand what's below it.

Because Laguz is the rune of water and therefore the moon, there are many ways to employ its magick in an effort to deepen one's connection with nature. One popular tool for magick is actually a combination of the two: moon water. Moon water is the product of leaving a bowl or clear receptacle of water out under the moon so that it may be charged with lunar energies. (It's best if it's from a natural source or filtered, but tap works, too.) It is recommended that the water be taken out of the sky's view before dawn. When making moon water, rainwater is my personal favorite to use. If it happens to rain *during* a full moon, this is a perfect time to collect.

The full moon is the typical phase to charge water, but one can choose different phases based on their magickal needs. I've made dark moon water by leaving water out under the moonless sky that occurs just before the new moon. Dark moon water works well for workings regarding death, endings, and pause. Waning moon water will support removal and minimization, while waxing will support growth and manifestation.

Once you have your own, keep it stored in a dark area. I keep my moon water in a glass decanter and place it on the windowsill or outside every full moon to increase the charge. This simple but powerful tool is great for consecrations, salt-water cleansings, flower essence bases, scrying, and really any magick that includes water. Add it to ritual baths or, if filtered water was used to make the moon water, use it to make tea and other beverages. If you happen to live in a part of the world that gets snow, I recommend collecting some in a jar and saving the melted water for magick. Snow water is ideal for purification.

The following is my personal recipe for Cleanse and Charge Spray, which I use to remove stagnant energetic residue from spaces or items while simultaneously imbuing them with uplifting energies:

❧ Cleanse and Charge Spray ☙

Ingredients:
>Moon water
>Snow water
>Vodka (to preserve)
>Mugwort
>Wormwood
>Angelica
>Hyssop
>Rosemary
>Labradorite chips
>Essential oils of rose, lavender, clary sage, and frankincense

How to Make

Add charged water to a kettle over low heat. Once the water begins to boil, remove from heat and immediately add your herbs. Let the water and herbs know their purpose in this blend and thank them for their aid in your magick. Keep the infusion covered and allow it to sit until it has cooled completely. Once the water is room temperature, strain out the herbs and add the water to a spray bottle with a small amount of vodka to preserve the mixture. Add the essential oils. Crystal chips are excellent additions to herbal sprays as well. Offer the discarded herbs to the Earth as a symbol of gratitude. If you don't have all the listed items, not to worry; these are simply the ingredients I prefer to use. Any cleansing and psychic herbs work just as well.

How to Use

During the dark or new moons phases I tend to perform "mass cleansings," which is where I gather all my magickal tools and clean them one by one. The Cleanse and Charge Spray can, of course, be used whenever it's needed, regardless of the astrological conditions. To use, spray the mixture directly on the item or on a clean towel. Wipe the item(s) clean while envisioning stagnant energies and psychic sludge disintegrating and transmuting. If using as a room spray, mist all four corners of the room beginning in the east corner and moving clockwise. If you'd like to speak an incantation or mantra during the cleansing, this is the time to do so. As the snow water, vodka, angelica, hyssop, and rosemary do the heavy-duty cleansing, the moon water, mugwort, wormwood, and labradorite simultaneously refresh and recharge with their energies. If it's a new or full moon, leave the cleansed items outside or on the windowsill overnight to soak up even more of that moon magick. Hail, Laguz!

CORRESPONDENCES OF LAGUZ

ELEMENT	Water
ZODIAC	Cancer, Pisces, Scorpio
PLANET	Moon
MOON PHASE	All
TAROT	The Moon, Queen of Cups
CRYSTAL	Celestite
CHAKRA	Third Eye
DEITIES	Chandra, Juturna, Mami Wata, Njord, Poseidon, Tefnut, Yemaya
PLANTS	Aloe, Bladderwrack, Butterfly Pea Blossom, Catnip, Hops, Jasmine, Violet, Willow

The plants of Laguz are deeply intuitive and emotional and comprise Divine Feminine energies. To get the most out of their magick, they are best employed on Mondays (which are ruled by the moon) or during the associated moon phase: waxing for gaining and increasing, waning for removing and decreasing, and full when strong energy is required.

Aloe
(*Aloe vera*)

Aloe resides under the rulership of Cancer and Scorpio and is therefore associated with the element of Water—a quality demonstrated by the gel within its leaves. This common houseplant nurtures and supports deep emotional healing. Drawing the Laguz stave over one's heart with the gel encourages opening and clearing of the heart chakra. True to the Water element, aloe is an ally for moon magick—particularly that of the dark moon phase. When performing Water magick, a combination of aloe, Laguz, and a Cancer or Scorpio moon will provide the ultimate energies to support such workings.

Medicinal Properties
The gel within aloe's leaves, which is 95 percent water and packed with vitamins, accelerates healing, and repairs damaged tissue. It is a well-known and effective cooling remedy for burns and other skin complaints. Aloe gel delays aging of the skin, treats dry conditions, fades scars like acne marks and stretch marks, heals cuts and bug bites, reduces infection risk, and soothes heat rash. It may be drunk daily as an immune-boosting supplement. Dab the gel on aching teeth or mouth ulcers. Combine with comfrey to treat fractures and broken bones. Actions: antibacterial, antifungal, anti-inflammatory, antioxidant, antiseptic, antiviral, demulcent, emollient, hepatic, laxative, purgative, rejuvenative, vermifuge, vulnerary. Cold and moistening.

Bladderwrack
(*Fucus vesiculosus*)

Bladderwrack is a seaweed that is often magickally applied to workings with water spirits and elementals. It is perfect as an offering to ocean deities. Its connection to water lends to dreamwork, sorting through complicated emotions, and the enhancement of psychic abilities. Enjoy as a hot tea or add to a ritual bath. Bladderwrack is associated with abundance and is ideal for money and career magick. Add to a floor wash for home or business to increase income. Bladderwrack offers protection to those traveling by water, especially when paired with Laguz and Elhaz.

Medicinal Properties

To reap the medicinal benefits of bladderwrack it is recommended that it be taken fresh. If that isn't possible, a powdered form is the next best thing. Because it is a demulcent, it does not work well in an alcohol tincture. Bladderwrack assists the body in nutrient assimilation and expels environmental toxins such as radiation. It supports healthy body weight and reduces excess hunger by stimulating the thyroid gland. It relieves acid reflux, lowers blood pressure, reduces an enlarged prostate, and speeds up the healing process post-illness. As an emollient, bladderwrack is nourishing for the hair and skin. As a compress, it treats rheumatic conditions, bruising, and sprains. Historically, it was used to treat tuberculosis. Actions: alterative, antibacterial, antibiotic, anticancer, anti-inflammatory, antioxidant, antirheumatic, demulcent, diuretic, emollient, expectorant, laxative, nutritive. Take regular breaks from use to support iodine balance. Cooling and moistening. Avoid alongside hyperthyroidism. Avoid during pregnancy and nursing.

Butterfly Pea Blossom
(*Clitoria ternatea*)

Butterfly pea blossom is a showstopper valued for its beauty as well as its many healing properties. Its suggestive shape is no doubt the inspiration for its Latin name and magickal connection to female sexuality and fertility. Butterfly pea blossom supports those on the path of spiritual transformation. We are able to see its physical transformative properties by simply adding citrus to an infusion, which alters the color from a vibrant indigo to a bright fuchsia—a display that reminds me of the raising from third eye to crown chakra. Butterfly pea blossom, which is associated with the moon, supports creativity and enhances psychic ability.

Medicinal Properties

Butterfly pea blossom is highly valued in ayurvedic and traditional Chinese medicine—and for good reasons! It is soothing and uplifting—a wonderful ally for those who suffer from anxiety and depression. As a nootropic plant, it supports cognitive health. Its bioflavonoids, antioxidant richness, and ability to stimulate collagen production fights premature aging of the skin and increases hair growth. Poor eyesight and glaucoma are improved by its ability to increase blood flow to the eyes. Butterfly pea blossom is an aphrodisiac that targets the female libido and treats vaginal complaints like leukorrhea. It lowers blood pressure and reduces fevers. Actions: analgesic, antibiotic, anticancer, anticonvulsive, anti-inflammatory, anxiolytic, antipyretic, diuretic, nootropic, sedative. Cooling.

Catnip
(*Nepeta cataria*)

For those with feline friends and familiars, catnip aids in strengthening the psychic connection between human and animal. While it is closely associated with cats, it works to strengthen the connection with any animal. As an offering, it's perfect for feline deities such as Bast, Sekhmet, Dawon, or even Freyja, whose chariot is pulled by two cats. In addition to animal magick, catnip is traditionally applied to love and fertility spells, money magick, and housewarming rituals. It is a mild hallucinatory and relaxant ideal for astral travel, dreamwork, divination, and shape-shifting—mainly in astral travel, but if you can shape shift outside of that, you win magick! Catnip helps to soothe nightmares, anxiety, and homesickness. It has a comforting motherly quality that works well for shadow work and trauma healing. Among all the magick you can employ it for, don't forget to add a few pinches to a small pouch for your cat—they will be quite appreciative!

Medicinal Properties

Catnip is a mild sedative with a cooling effect. It treats several issues such as colds, insomnia, hysteria, nervous headaches, nervous stomach, and delayed menstruation. It even repels insects! For children, it helps to soothe hyperactivity, teething pain, colic, fever, diarrhea, and indigestion. It should not, however, be given to children for extended periods of time. Small doses of the herb should be administered to avoid stomach upset and vomiting. Catnip is an excellent addition to calming massage oils. Dab the infusion on eyes to relieve swelling and puffiness. When making tea or tinctures with catnip, the fresh plant is best. Actions: anodyne, antispasmodic, astringent, bronchodilator, carminative, diaphoretic, digestive, emmenagogue, febrifuge, hemostatic, nervine, refrigerant, sedative, stimulant. Cooling and drying. Avoid during pregnancy and nursing. Avoid alongside alcohol and sedative pharmaceuticals.

Hops
(*Humulus lupulus*)

Hops grow on a climbing vine and are best known as a major ingredient in beer. In magick, they are common allies for visionary work and lucid dreaming. Create a prophetic dreams spell bottle with hops and other herbs such as catnip, lavender, mugwort, and vervain. Label the bottle with the Laguz rune and keep it beside or beneath the bed. Refresh the contents when necessary. Add the flowers to a pre-bedtime bath to encourage restful deep sleep and to floor washes to help deter chaos from the home.

Medicinal Properties

Hops provide beer with its famous bitter flavor, and it's the familiar bitterness of this herb that stimulates healthy digestion. Its potent nervine and sedative qualities help soothe anxiety, insomnia, and irritability. Hops cleanse the blood and organs, enhance the production of breastmilk, increase sex drive in women, and decrease sex drive in men. Drink a cup of hops tea before a meal to reduce bloating and excessive gas. Hops are good for rashes, bruises, and sprains. Actions: analgesic, antacid, antispasmodic, anxiolytic, bitter, digestive, diuretic, estrogenic, galactagogue, nervine, sedative, soporific, stomachic, vulnerary. Cooling. Those who suffer from depression should avoid hops. If pregnant, consult with a healthcare professional before using.

Jasmine
(*Jasminum grandiflorum*)

Jasmine is a mildly euphoric lunar flower that is associated with moon goddesses such as Artemis, Chang'e, Diana, or Rhiannon, as well as the Divine Feminine. Its sensuality lends to beauty, love, and sex magick. Wearing the scent is said to bring true love. Jasmine amplifies spell work and offers psychic protection. It works to clear the aura of stagnant and harmful energies. The flowers are perfect for cleansing and charging crystals, tarot cards, and runes. The essential oil is calming and stress-relieving and when added to a diffuser, aids in meditation and trance work. Keep dried bundles in the home to promote a peaceful environment. Dab a small, diluted amount of jasmine oil on the third eye before divination and astral magick.

Medicinal Properties

Jasmine is a calming flower that eases depression, anxiety, and irritability. It stimulates the production of dopamine in the brain. Dab jasmine infusion on irritated eyes to relieve them. Topically, the flower oil moisturizes, enhances elasticity, soothes sunburn, and treats dermatitis. It relieves muscle spasms and soreness. Jasmine's light floral aroma is uplifting and beneficial for those who suffer from depression, chronic stress, and anxiety. As an emmenagogue, jasmine eases menstrual pain. The flower essence is recommended for those who have trouble sleeping or have high-strung type A personalities. Actions: antidepressant, anxiolytic, antiseptic, antispasmodic, aromatic, emmenagogue, nervine, sedative, vulnerary. Warming and moistening.

Violet
(*Viola* spp.)

Those who are grieving will find comfort in the gentle and nurturing energies of violets. Traditionally the flowers have been strewn over graves to honor passed loved ones. These harbingers of springtime are associated with renewal, love, and the Ostara sabbat. They bring good fortune to women, and because they are associated with feminine beauty, the dried flowers are ideal for burning during glamour magick. The blossoms make appropriate offerings when working with goddesses of the moon. Combine violets with roses or jasmine flowers for spells to attract a romantic partner. To increase intuition, make a cup of violet tea; use a teaspoon or finger (if it's not too hot) to trace the Laguz rune on the surface of the liquid. As you do this, imagine Laguz charging the tea with the powers of intuition, which then transfer to you as you enjoy your beverage.

Medicinal Properties

Violets are cooling and moistening flowers great for dry conditions such as constipation and dry cough. They detox the body, strengthen immunity, and cleanse the blood. The anti-inflammatory qualities are mildly pain relieving and help to soothe joint pain and arthritis. The flowers help with skin conditions like rashes and insect bites. Use as a salve, poultice, or skin wash for skin irritations. Violets make safe and gentle laxatives for children. In the Middle East, Iran in particular, violet oil is a traditional remedy for insomnia. Actions: alterative, analgesic, antibacterial, anti-inflammatory, antiseptic, demulcent, diaphoretic, emetic, expectorant, febrifuge, laxative. Cooling and moistening. The roots and seeds are toxic, do not ingest.

Willow
(*Salix* spp.)

The sight of a weeping willow is enough to stir emotion. It's a tree of magnificence, yet there's a sorrow to it as well—hence the name. The moon and Water element, which are inextricably tied to emotion, rule over willows. The tree is typically found in graveyards to comfort those who are grieving and to ward off evil. Willows harness incredible magick and are applied to workings of intuition, psychic ability, dreamwork, love, healing, lunar and feminine magick, conjuring, and protection. Those who are looking to attract love should carry the leaves on their person while out and about. When searching for a lost object, call on willow's psychic powers to help track it down. The wood, which has long been used for the construction of witches' besoms, is ideal for making runes and wands. If you happen upon already broken branches, a Laguz talisman can be easily made with some twine and placed above a doorway in the home as a reminder of one's connection to the divine. The synergy of Laguz and willow trees creates an immense psychic magick perfect for moon and water rituals, feminine magick, and divination. The two go together like black cats and Halloween, or like lamb and tuna fish. (Big Daddy, anyone?)

Medicinal Properties

Willow bark, also known as witches' aspirin, contains the compound salicin, which is a natural reliever for pain, fever, and inflammation. It's effective for backaches, migraines, and rheumatic pain. Unlike aspirin, however, it does not thin the blood. Combine with St. John's wort to treat nerve pain. Willow's cooling properties aid in the relief of the hot flashes and night sweats that often occur during menopause. It helps to restore vitality in weak conditions. Actions: alterative, analgesic, anaphrodisiac, anodyne, antibacterial, anti-inflammatory, antiseptic, antirheumatic, astringent, diaphoretic, digestive, sedative. Cooling and drying. Those who are allergic to aspirin should avoid willow. Avoid during pregnancy. Avoid long-term use.

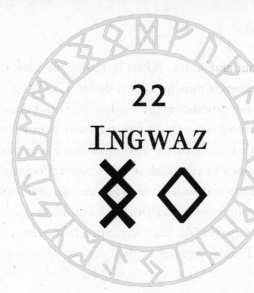

22
INGWAZ

Phonetic equivalent: ing
Seed, Development, Male Fertility

Ingwaz is the single seed
Buried in cold dark soil
From which the seedling rises
It reaches for the Sun

Ingwaz, or Inguz, which has a sound value of "ing," is an Earth element rune that symbolizes seeds and fertility. It is named for the old god Ing who is likely synonymous with the Vanir god Freyr. As a Vanir god, Freyr rules over gold, prosperity, and virility. He is often depicted with an erect penis to indicate his role as a fertility deity. Ingwaz is sexual and masculine in nature and is counter to the feminine Perthro. Like Teiwaz, the seed rune is a symbol of the Divine Masculine.

Ingwaz symbolizes potential, growth, channeling energy, personal development, and the male procreative force (seeds sperm). Note how one version of the rune stave resembles DNA, the building blocks that contain the unique blueprints for every living being. The second version of the Ingwaz stave resembles a seed, which germinates and becomes the harvest of Jera. Notice how the shape of the Jera stave is merely an open version of Ingwaz. Together Ingwaz and Jera harness the energy of a life cycle. Ingwaz is generally a beneficial and fruitful rune, and there are no reverse or murkstave meanings.

In magick the shape of the seed rune is regarded and used as a portal to the *other worlds* much like a hag stone or the opening of a well. It is a gateway to the nine worlds of the Yggdrasil tree. For those who work with Hekate, Ingwaz works well as a magickal representation of the crossroads—a meeting point of liminal boundaries. Pair with Ehwaz, the vehicle rune, to ensure a smooth journey out of the physical realm.

The presence of Ingwaz in a reading typically indicates a period of potential and growth. With Ehwaz, it may indicate a blossoming romance. When paired with Uruz it can point to the onset of a healing journey.

Ingwaz is the idea that precedes every invention, every creation, and every action. It's behind the technological advancement of the human race. When the Earth is viewed from space, we are able to see the vast green expanse of our forests and grasslands clearly. Of all life on Earth trees are dominant by far, as scientists estimate there are just over three trillion. Every single one is a product of Ingwaz. Every towering tree that provides wood for our homes, furniture, and the paper of this book, they are all results of seeds—the microcosm that holds the blueprint of the macrocosm. Just as the tiny acorn encompasses the mighty oak, so does Ingwaz encompass the entire physical world around us.

Ingwaz connects us to nature through the cultivation of our own gardens or collection of indoor plants. Mother Nature is the backbone of witchcraft—the raison d'être. What exactly is it about the natural world that makes our hearts so full? Nature is unapologetically authentic, enchantingly wild, and full of limitless magick. To some, including myself, unadulterated nature is synonymous with what many call *God*.

Before writing this section today, I took advantage of the gorgeous weather and hiked some trails I'd never taken before. While being technically part of the city, the park air smelled clean and fresh, and the surrounding greenery transported me to a whole different place. Being alone in a forest is one of the few instances when I can get out of my head with ease and be perfectly mindful. I walked slowly, absorbing my surroundings while speaking silent words of gratitude. At one point I felt so free and at peace I almost cried. I know many can relate to this feeling.

Having gardens and/or indoor plants is our way of bringing small pieces of Mother Nature to our homes. When I first became a "plant mom" I was discouraged by my lack of a green thumb. All my plants eventually died—even the ones people recommended to me because they are "difficult to kill." Difficult, schmifficult—I was an unstoppable serial killer of plants. Like anything, however, we learn from our mistakes, from the advice of others, and from research. I'm happy to report that (most of) my plants thrive these days! Even though I'd taken courses on herbalism, such courses don't necessarily teach you how to cultivate your own plants.

If you can relate to my previous plant-parenting troubles, keep in mind that adding plants to your space doesn't mean you have to start from seeds. Home improvement stores, farmers markets, and nurseries offer a wide selection of garden ready plants, herbs, and veggies. Just like immersing yourself in nature, adorning the home with indoor plants comes with many benefits. Studies* have shown that interacting with them by repotting or pruning, for example, can reduce blood pressure and general stress. Horticultural therapy has been used to relieve anxiety and depression while promoting a sense of well-being. Whether you're in a forest or surrounded by potted greenery in your home, researchers have found improved outlooks as well as improved air quality. The best plants for indoor air freshening are rubber trees, spider plants, Boston ferns, and ficus trees.

When choosing indoor plants there are a few things to consider. If you have pets or young children, you'll want to choose varieties that are nontoxic. Poison control centers offer resources and lists of toxic plants. Maintenance is another consideration. You'll want to know how much sunlight a plant needs and whether it needs to be direct. Most potted plants that can be purchased come with small informational cards that provide directions on watering and sunlight requirements. Because of the large oak in my front yard, half of my house does not get a lot of sunlight. As a result, I keep most of my indoor plants in the back of my home where the late afternoon sun has access to them. I found that starting with

---

*Min-sun Lee, Juyoung Lee, Bum-Jin Park, and Yoshifumi Miyazaki, "Interaction with Indoor Plants May Reduce Psychological and Physiological Stress by Suppressing Autonomic Nervous System Activity in Young Adults: A Randomized Crossover Study," *Journal of Physiological Anthropology* 34, no. 1 (2015): 21.

indoor plants was a wonderful segue into beginning an outdoor garden.

If, like me, you live in the city, you may wonder if an outdoor garden is even possible for you. My "backyard" is a rooftop, and on it I keep a raised garden bed that a friend built for me with scrap wood. It measures six feet by five feet, and while that may seem small, I am currently growing romaine lettuce, broccoli, peas, tomatoes, basil, and lavender with room to spare! Not bad for a small wooden rectangle filled with dirt. Also, most cities these days offer community garden space for those who can't grow at home, and a quick internet search will let you know where you can find the ones nearest to you.

In chapter 4 we discussed communicating with plants and being able to work hands on with them is a wonderful precursor to eventual interaction. Working hands on provides a sturdy foundation on which a meaningful relationship can be built. If having a garden is just not possible for you, having even one small potted plant is enough to initiate a personal relationship to the green world. If you are anything like I was, though, and tend to end up with dead plants, maybe start with something low maintenance like a succulent (which includes cacti and aloe) or a spider plant. If you find that your plants keep dying, don't give up; find out what went wrong, talk to plant people, do some research, and trust that a little practice goes a long way. Hail, Ingwaz!

CORRESPONDENCES OF INGWAZ

ELEMENT	Earth
ZODIAC	Aquarius
PLANET	Mars, Jupiter
MOON PHASE	New Moon, Waxing
TAROT	The Emperor, King of Cups
CRYSTAL	Pyrite
CHAKRA	Root
DEITIES	Äkräs, Cernunnos, Freyr, Lono, Pan, Priapus
PLANTS	Black Cohosh, Blessed Thistle, Mistletoe, Pine, Saw Palmetto

The plants of Ingwaz represent the metaphorical planting of seeds, nurturing, and growth. They are ideal in magickal workings regarding new ideas, otherworldly travel, fertility, and virility.

Black Cohosh
(*Cimicifuga racemosa*)

Traditionally black cohosh, also known as black snake root, is an aggressive remedy for impotence and was often added to wine or to ritual baths to increase libido and fertility. Black cohosh and Ingwaz combined result in potent male sexual energy. To commence a fertility ritual, add a bit of powdered plant to red wine (or grape juice for those who abstain from alcohol) and trace the Ingwaz stave on the fluid's surface nine times before taking a drink. Black cohosh also works to keep evil at bay and can be sprinkled around the entryways of the home or added to floor washes to increase protection—especially if one suspects they're under psychic attack.

Medicinal Properties

Black cohosh is commonly used to help ease the symptoms of menopause such as hot flashes, mood fluctuations, vaginal dryness, and night sweats. It helps to relieve dysmenorrhea and treat polycystic ovary syndrome. Black cohosh can help alleviate asthma, severe cough, and cold. It is an effective remedy against high blood pressure, tinnitus, and arthritis pain and improves circulation. Actions: alterative, analgesic, antidepressant, anti-inflammatory, antirheumatic, antispasmodic, antivenomous, digestive, emmenagogue, expectorant, estrogenic, hypotensive, sedative. Avoid during pregnancy and nursing. Cooling. Avoid large doses as it may cause headache, dizziness, and nausea. Avoid alongside liver problems.

Blessed Thistle
(*Cnicus benedictus* or *Carduus benedictus*)

Blessed thistle is a martial herb of protection, strength, and men's mysteries. As an offering, it is ideal for spirits who watch over nature and wildlife. It is particularly sacred to the horned gods Cernunnos and Pan. Blessed thistle represents potent sexuality and may be used for the invoking of fertility gods such as Freyr. As an aphrodisiac, it is well suited for sex magick. If you are a target of ill will or a curse, blessed thistle will work to not only block the harmful energy but also return it to the sender. Blessed thistle and Ingwaz paired are a fierce duo for fertility and Divine Masculine magick.

Medicinal Properties

Blessed thistle facilitates healthy digestion, stimulates the appetite, and supports liver function. As an expectorant, it works to thin mucus resulting in a more productive cough. Although mostly thought of as an herb for men's health, blessed thistle is a galactagogue, which means it increases the production of the breastmilk—it is, however, not to be confused with milk thistle. In the Middle Ages it was believed to be a cure for the plague. Action: alterative, antibacterial, antifungal, anti-inflammatory, bitter, cholagogue, expectorant, galactagogue, emetic, hepatic, vulnerary. Cooling and drying. Avoid during pregnancy. Large doses may cause vomiting. It is not recommended as an incense as the smoke may cause irritation of the sinuses and throat.

Mistletoe
(*Viscum album*)

Mistletoe is a parasitic plant that makes its home on various trees. Many are familiar with mistletoe; some of us have even kissed beneath it. It was sacred to the ancient Druids who referred to it as "all healer." The Druids believed that happening upon the plant indicated the presence of the gods. It represents love, creativity, and fertility and may be worn to help a couple conceive. Mistletoe is a strongly protective plant that can be placed throughout the home to protect the family at any time—not just Yule! It is suggested that in its presence, ghosts cannot hide and evil cannot dwell. Mistletoe is perfect for love spells, particularly when there is a specific person of desire. In Norse mythology, it is associated with the god Baldur, son of Odin and Frigga. When Baldur was born, Frigga beseeched all the world's beings to never harm her child, which in turn made him invincible—but she overlooked mistletoe. Eventually, Baldur meets his demise when he is struck by an arrow containing the plant. In Old Norse tradition it was said that if one encountered an enemy beneath the mistletoe, both parties were to lay down their weapons and interact peacefully; from this evolved the current tradition of kissing beneath the mistletoe, transforming the plant from a symbol of hate and death to one of love and life.

Medicinal Properties

Historically, mistletoe was used to treat seizures, tinnitus, vertigo, and hypertension but has fallen out of modern medicinal use due to its toxicity. Actions: cardiac, emmenagogue, hypotensive, nervine, relaxant, sedative. Cooling and drying. Mistletoe is somewhat toxic and may be safely used by adults in small amounts under the supervision of a healthcare professional. For animals and children, mistletoe can result in death. Always avoid during pregnancy and nursing.

Pine
(*Pinus* spp.)

Like mistletoe, pine is a symbol of Yule, Christmas, and other winter traditions. Today many of us know it best as the "Christmas tree." This practice arose from the pre-Christian tradition of bringing evergreen boughs into the home during the winter holidays—a symbolic act of preservation since pines thrive in winter while the majority of plants reach the end of their life cycles. The boughs were also believed to bring about protection from starvation and illness. The dried needles and resin of the tree may be added to incense to assist in the cleansing of a space, and perhaps this is the reason pine is often added to so many commercial household cleaners. That and its uplifting fresh scent, of course. The pine tree is associated with male sexuality, and the cones especially make great talismans for fertility magick. It exudes vibes of positivity, health, and confidence. This coniferous tree has a hospitable energy and is ideal for décor and incense during gatherings. Magickally, pine can aid one in uncovering the truth.

Medicinal Properties

Pine bark works well in clearing congestion and wet coughs and is ideal for chronic lung and sinus infections. The inner bark contains vitamin C and has been used to shorten the duration of colds and flu. When the tell-tale signs of cold and flu begin, combine with elderberry for a tea that can be taken daily while symptoms persist. Pine pitch helps to heal wounds and soothe sores, boils, rashes, and burns. The essential oil aids in calming stress and anger. Add it to massage oil to alleviate sore muscles. The pollen, which contains testosterone, aids men who are unable to naturally produce enough of the hormone. Actions: antiseptic, aromatic, expectorant, testosterone-enhancing, vulnerary. Warming and drying.

Saw Palmetto
(*Sabal serrulata, Serenoa repens*)

Saw palmetto is energetically masculine, associated with Mars and the element of Fire. Magickally, it may be used to assist a man in gaining a desired lover and increase sexual energy. To reap its aphrodisiacal qualities, it's common practice to add the berries of saw palmetto to alcoholic beverages such as wine. This is a suitable herb for those who work with the Norse god Freyr who, among other things, is the god of virility; this is made quite clear in the depictions of Freyr sporting a large erect penis. Saw palmetto is best used magickally on Tuesdays (day of Mars and Tyr) and works to invoke the assertive energies and virtues of the planet and/or corresponding deities.

Medicinal Properties
Saw palmetto is supportive of men's health, effectively treating ailments such as prostatitis, prostate cancer, and urinary problems. Elderly men, particularly those who suffer from wasting conditions, can benefit from regular use. Saw palmetto promotes digestive health and weight gain. The roots and leaves may be used as a remedy for dysentery. The berries are effective against severe coughs. They are also used in treating hair loss caused by alopecia. Saw palmetto may delay menopause in women. Actions: anti-inflammatory, antispasmodic, digestive, diuretic, expectorant, sedative, tonic. Warming and moistening. Avoid while nursing.

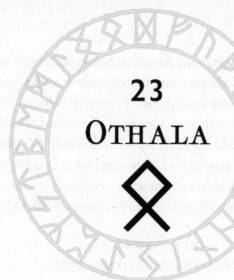

23
OTHALA

Phonetic equivalent: O
Home, Family, Ancestors

Othala's where the heart resides
A place of shelter, love, and rest
Built with bones and blood of ancestors
Upon this land we're safe and blessed

Othala is the rune of home and family. In this book it is the second to last rune, but it's not uncommon to see Futhark sequences in which it is the final rune. There is debate about whether Othala or Dagaz should finalize the Elder Futhark; I personally subscribe to Dagaz as the final rune, and I will present my reasons in the following chapter. There is also an Uthark theory in which Uruz is the first rune and Fehu is the twenty-fourth; however, that is beyond the scope of this book.

Basic meanings for Othala include ancestral heritage and wisdom, property, tradition, and sanctuary. It represents general inheritance—of land, belief systems, and genetics as well as one's fundamental values, sense of belonging, and connection to familial roots. In its simplicity, it is a place where one feels safe and accepted.

Energetically, the ancestor rune has the power to invoke the god Odin, much like Ansuz. It lends its talents to past life work, the healing of family traumas, and honoring and communicating with ancestors.

In a reading, Othala may be pointing out that one's current situation is directly affected by their upbringing. It may also suggest the need to reach out to loved ones for support *or* to offer support to a loved one who is currently struggling. Another possibility is that it is asking you to challenge learned belief systems that only serve to hold you back. If it presents itself in a reading alongside Dagaz, it may illustrate a change within the dynamics of a family or household. With Berkana, a reading possibly refers to a mother figure or pregnancy. Reversed, it can indicate displacement, lack of security, loss of possessions, enduring family trauma, family conflict, or homelessness.

Based on its shape and meaning, this rune appears to be a combination of Gebo and Ingwaz and resembles DNA like Ingwaz as well. One may also consider Othala the rune that represents the physical living body—the sacred temple that houses the spirit. Like the walls of one's home, it offers comfort and shielded protection from the harshness and uncertainty of the outside world. In regard to the Yggdrasill tree and the nine worlds among it, this rune represents Midgard, or Earth. Like Mannaz, Othala is the tribe, which may be blood family, a coven, or any group of people working in tandem toward the same goal. Othala's shape may be used to gather and seal in energy, similar to that of knot magick.

Othala keeps us connected to our roots, both familial and of the Earth. By tapping into the power of ancestral connection, we can honor and commune with nature as those before us did. Exploring our ancestry has never been easier with the popularity of DNA testing kits. DNA testing is especially helpful for those who have no other way of knowing their blood roots, such as those who were adopted at birth.

When it comes to ancestry, however, the concept is not limited to blood relation. Those who practice within the occult arts may choose to view magickal predecessors as ancestors, regardless of blood relation. The only right way is what feels right for you.

My personal practice is rather eclectic due to my eclectic heritage. I'm mostly southern Italian but I also have Irish roots, Scandinavian, Egyptian, Middle Eastern, Iberian, and Balkan—and I've found that I'm innately drawn to these particular cultures of spirituality. My practice is heavily influenced by Italian folk magick, Celtic spirituality, Norse magick and mythology, ancient Egyptian mythology, Buddhism, and Balkan traditions. I study these traditions and explore them through meditation and inner journeying. I call upon ancestors of blood as well as ancestors of magick, depending on the situation or the knowledge I'm seeking.

One thing we know for sure is that our ancient ancestors were at the constant mercy of nature and in turn did their best to honor and appease the land, air, and water spirits. Today many of us don't worry about food shortages during droughts or blizzards, as we have the luxury of local markets and grocery stores. It is the luxuries that we depend on today that have yielded an unfortunate disconnect between the modern human and the wildness of Earth. Don't get me wrong; I'm not complaining about luxuries. I can't imagine the difficulties that accompanied basic survival for those long before us. Whether they wanted it or not, closeness to nature was not optional—it was just reality. There was no separation from it. Many of us today do have a choice regarding how big a role nature will play in our lives.

If you're not sure how to incorporate the nature connection into your life, you can look to the ancestors for guidance. For me, incorporating the connection might mean choosing days in which I spend all my free time outdoors, only eating foods from my garden, or forgoing technological conveniences. When harvesting food and herbs from my garden, I feel a strong connection to my ancestors, specifically my Italian ancestors; perhaps that's due to the potent smell of all my basil!

Studying and working with symbols is also a practice I use to sense and build ancestral connections. Besides the obvious runes, I work with Icelandic staves such as the *vegvisir,* the Egyptian ankh, and eyes of Horus and Ra, the Celtic triquetra, and the Eastern Aum symbol, among many others. Symbols unlock a primal way of thinking and are the brain's shortcuts to otherwise complicated meanings. Meditating with or even simply studying a symbol from your lineage is a great way to initiate a relationship with those who came before you.

Othala is an ally for rewilding because it is a magickal representation of the home all of us share—the Earth. Therefore, there's no better rune to ask: What can my ancestors teach me about what it means to truly be a part of the natural world? You don't have to ditch your house, job, car, and other belongings and go live in a small shack in the forest to live a life close to nature. We can live in our modern world with our modern technologies while making time for the outdoors to keep our spirits firmly rooted to the Earth. Hail, Othala!

CORRESPONDENCES OF OTHALA

ELEMENT	Earth
ZODIAC	Taurus
PLANET	Jupiter
MOON PHASE	Full
TAROT	10 of Pentacles
CRYSTAL	Peridot
CHAKRA	Heart
DEITIES	Bes, Brigid, Chantico, Frigga, Hestia, Zao Jun
PLANTS	Avens, Bayberry, Blackberry, Coriander, Vervain, Vetiver, Witch Hazel

The plants of Othala represent ancestral connection and the energies that we wish to invite into our homes and families. These plants aid in magickal workings regarding our heritage, protection of home and family, tradition, and the breaking of generational traumas.

Avens
(*Geum urbanum*)

Herbalist Maud Grieve suggests that avens has been called the "blessed herb" and was believed to "ward off evil spirits and venomous beasts."[*] She also notes that *The Hortus Sanitatis,* printed in 1491, states "Where the root is in the house, Satan can do nothing and flies from it." From

---

*Maud Grieve, "Avens," Botanical.com, 2021.

this we can surmise that avens is quite useful for cleansings and exorcisms. The dried, powdered root may be added to incense blends and burned when a space needs hefty fumigation. When engaging in potentially dangerous magick such as necromancy, create a barrier circle of powdered avens, frankincense, and angelica as a protective shield from harmful energies. The circle should be large enough to contain the practitioner as well as any ritual tools needed.

Medicinal Properties

Avens is often used for its astringent qualities; it treats mouth sores, diarrhea, and irritable bowel syndrome. Topically it may be used to relieve hemorrhoids and to help reduce or altogether stop excessive bleeding. It may be used as a fever reducer. Actions: anti-inflammatory, antiseptic, astringent, diaphoretic, febrifuge, styptic. Drying. Currently, there is not enough research to support if avens is safe during pregnancy—err on the side of caution and avoid during pregnancy and nursing.

Bayberry
(*Myrica cerifera*)

The root of bayberry, or wax myrtle as it's also called, has been used in North American folk traditions for house blessings, increasing luck, and money-drawing spells. It has strong domestic vibes and an affinity for the home. Bayberry is ruled by Jupiter, the planet of good fortune and growth. Wax from the berries may be used to make candles and soaps and is a vegan substitute for beeswax. When a debt is left unpaid, the magick of bayberry is said to ensure the return of the money owed. Add the dried roots, leaves, or berries to incense for home blessings and cleansings. If your house happens to be inhabited by ghosts, bayberry incense and ritual can be employed to gently help them find peace and move on.

Medicinal Properties

Medicinally, bayberry is quite similar to avens; it's strongly astringent, which is beneficial in treating gastrointestinal distress such as diarrhea, colitis, and dysentery. As a mild stimulant, it increases circulation. The powdered root is recommended for cold and flu symptoms, especially sore throat and fever. As a topical salve, bayberry helps to relieve muscle and joint pain. Actions: antibacterial, astringent, emetic, expectorant, hemostatic, stimulant, styptic, vulnerary. Warming and drying. Bayberry should not be taken in large doses or long term due to its level of astringency. Avoid during pregnancy.

Blackberry
(*Rubus fruticosus*)

According to Mrs. Grieve, Blackberries offer protection against all "evil runes" if gathered under the "right moon phase."[*] It does not mention *which* moon phase, but I was much more intrigued by the *evil runes* part. Here I should again mention that no single rune is inherently "bad" or "evil," but they may absolutely be used in cursing and hexing. We know that what makes certain magick evil is the intent of the practitioner. I should also include here that the word *rune,* which translates to "secret" in Proto-Germanic, is not exclusive to the ancient Germanic alphabets. Blackberry's ability to ward off evil is perfect for general home protection and magick against psychic attacks. The thorns particularly may be employed in defensive magick; therefore, blackberry is also a valued companion for Thurisaz. For a quick and easy home protection charm, glue multiple Blackberry thorns to a piece of paper in the shape of Othala and place it near the main entrance(s) of the home. If extra protection is needed add Othala to a bindrune with Elhaz and Thurisaz, and if necessary, notify the proper authorities in the case of danger!

Medicinal Properties

Blackberry root is one of the most effective astringents in relieving wet cough, mouth sores, sore throats, diarrhea, and dysentery to name a few. It is a gentle (and delicious) remedy for children suffering from diarrhea. Sore eyes may be soothed with the compresses of diluted tea. Blackberries are vitamin and mineral rich and helpful in treating ane-

---

[*]Maud Grieve, "Blackberry," Botanical.com, 2021.

mia. Add blackberry and witch hazel to a bath to treat hemorrhoids. Actions: anti-inflammatory, antioxidant, astringent, nutritive. Cooling and drying.

Coriander
(*Coriandrum sativum*)

Coriander, also known as cilantro and Chinese parsley, is said to bring peace and protection to the gardener that grows it. Hang dried bunches in doorways to invite peaceful energies into the home while repelling chaos and harmful energies. Coriander helps to repel illness and encourage a speedy healing process for those who are sick. It is an aphrodisiac and may be used in love, sex, and fertility magick. In certain traditions of Chinese mysticism, it has been used it to create love potions and enhance one's quality of life.

Medicinal Properties
Coriander is a strong detoxifier. It remedies coughs, bloating, excessive gas, and digestive cramps. Coriander helps to quell anxiety, tension, and nervousness and bring on sleep. Apply topically to soothe rheumatic pain. Because it helps strengthen the urinary tract, those who suffer from chronic infections would benefit from regular use. Actions: aphrodisiac, aromatic, carminative, diaphoretic, diuretic, expectorant, nervine. Cooling and drying.

Vervain
(*Verbena officinalis*)

Vervain is such a magickally versatile herb, it would honestly work well aside just about any rune. I've included it with Othala because it of its ability to repel that which we don't want in our homes (e.g., curses and malefic energies) while attracting the things we do want such as wealth, spiritual and physical wellness, and love. It may be used to bless, heal, protect, purify. As a potent visionary herb, vervain assists in connecting one to spirits, the underworld, and the infinite mysteries of the cosmos. It aids practitioners in the honing of their divination skills. It works to reverse curses and hexes and should be worn during exorcisms. Druids employed it to purify and consecrate sacred spaces and to contact the land spirits. It is said that Vervain is most potent when collected during Litha, the summer solstice. Add it to any magickal charm to amplify the power of a spell. It inspires creativity and is considered an "artist's herb." Keep a bundle in an infant's room (but out of their reach!) to add reinforcements of general protection. Vervain is said to have been used to cleanse the crucifixion wounds of Jesus.

Medicinal Properties

Vervain is just as multitalented in medicine as it is with magick. It is used to reduce swelling, spasms, and convulsions. As a poultice around the shoulders, neck, and nape, it alleviates tension and headaches that result. It is an ideal cooling remedy for "hot" conditions like inflammation, irritability, and anger. Vervain restores the nervous system and promotes healthy digestion. It makes a great tonic for those recovering from addiction and/or chronic illness. It helps prevent and dissolve kidney and gallstones. Actions: mild antidepressant, antispasmodic, anxiolytic, mild bitter, cholagogue, diaphoretic, digestive, emmenagogue, febrifuge, galactagogue, hepatic, nervine, rubefacient, tonic, vermifuge. Cooling and drying. Large doses may cause vomiting. Avoid during pregnancy. Avoid alongside anticoagulants and mineral supplements.

Vetiver
(*Vetiveria zizanioides*)

Vetiver is repellant of all entities with ill intentions, especially those that wish to take what doesn't belong to them. Keep in the home or vehicle to protect the people and items inside. It's especially helpful for businesses as it repels thieves while simultaneously attracting customers and financial success. The incense smoke and essential oil may be used to refresh the energies of divinatory tools. It is useful for emotional wellness magick, grounding, and shielding. Vetiver aids in settling disputes among arguing family members, friends, or romantic partners.

Medicinal Properties

Vetiver is mainly used as an essential oil to promote relaxation while lifting one's spirits. Like Othala, vetiver is ruled by the grounding element of Earth and is therefore deeply balancing and calming. Those who suffer from nighttime restlessness can benefit from its tranquil energies. When added to skincare products, vetiver oil helps to firm, tighten, and protect the skin from environmental damage. Its natural cooling abilities make vetiver oil a great topical for the uncomfortable heat of fever. Actions: anti-inflammatory, antioxidant, antiseptic, aphrodisiac, cicatrizant, nervine, refrigerant, sedative, vulnerary.

Witch Hazel
(*Hamamelis virginiana*)

Magickally, witch hazel may be used in the form of dowsing rods for finding lost items or treasures in the Earth. It works to heal broken hearts, especially after a complicated breakup. Burn witch hazel or add to a floor wash to protect the home and family against evil influences. If you live in a heavily populated area, keep some of the plant in your pocket to protect your auric health from being influenced by others. Witch hazel contains the energies of the sun and fire and is ideal for drawing love, passion, and vitality into the home.

Medicinal Properties

Witch hazel is a versatile astringent primarily used as an ingredient in skincare products. Apply topically to relieve inflammation and pain and to staunch bleeding. It is suitable for colds and respiratory infections that produce a lot of mucus. Add to sitz baths to treat hemorrhoids or apply as an eyewash to alleviate inflammation. Witch hazel soothes excess itching and a variety of skin conditions such as eczema, cysts, and tumors. Like many other astringent herbs, it is useful for relieving diarrhea. Witch hazel may be used as a post-abortion tonic. Actions: analgesic, anti-inflammatory, astringent, sedative, styptic, vulnerary. Neutral and drying. Use internally only under the guidance of a healthcare professional. Never ingest during pregnancy and nursing.

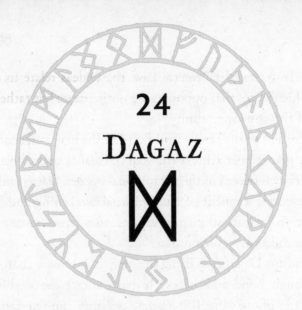

24

DAGAZ

Phonetic equivalent: D
Daybreak, Transformation, Enlightenment

Dagaz is infinity
Where dark becomes the light
Where day becomes the night
And on and on it goes . . .

We made it. Dagaz (pronounced dag-ahz) marks the end of the Elder Futhark. The final rune translates to *daylight,* but more specifically, it refers to *twilight,* the liminal phase between darkness and sunrise. Thus, it's a rune of breakthrough and transformation.

As the final rune of the Elder Futhark, it may be thought of as an ending, but like the dark moon phase, it is merely a period of transition and rebirth. Its shape, which is similar to the infinity symbol, indicates a lack of beginning or end; it is in constant motion like a pendulum. As the final rune, it refers to reaching the ultimate state of spiritual awakening, sometimes referred to as enlightenment.

Dagaz represents polarities and the reconciliation of opposites. During the process of the spiritual awakening, one is able to reconcile the material body with the subtle spirit, the feminine with the masculine, and the above with the below. The illusions of duality are replaced with cohesive understanding and unconditional acceptance of cosmic

242

wholeness. In terms of Hermetic Law, these ideas relate to the law of polarity, which states that opposites are not separate but rather contrasting ends of the same spectrum.

Dagaz relates to the tarot's world card of the major arcana. Both seek to help the practitioner achieve the goal of balance and wholeness—two concepts clearly reflected in their traditional images. Dagaz and the world card illustrate the moment of true spiritual awakening and loss of ego attachment. In their most spiritual aspects, they represent unity with the cosmos and collective consciousness.

In a reading, Dagaz may bring the news of immense change coming, a breakthrough, hope, and success. It may indicate the need for balance within an area of one's life. It is a very auspicious rune containing forces that may be evoked to work in one's favor. When drawn alongside Fehu, the reading may be highlighting that a career change is necessary. With Elhaz it may represent a pivotal time in one's spiritual journey. Dagaz cannot be murkstave, although its radically transformational energies can surely blindside an unsuspecting party.

In the following paragraphs, I will explain why I prefer the Elder Futhark sequence in which Dagaz is the final rune. Dagaz is the twenty-fourth rune, relating to the twenty-four hours in a day, while its counterpart Jera is the twelfth rune (half of twenty-four) and relates to the twelve months in a year. Jera is the yearly cycle and Dagaz is the daily cycle. Jera is gentle, slow change while Dagaz is swift, absolute change.

I believe, regarding the cycle of the runes, Jera and Dagaz are meant to be counterparts, which would not be possible if Othala took the final position. When the Elder Futhark is written out in a circle, Dagaz and Jera are in direct opposition of one another. Beyond that, as a rune of radical transformation, its place at the end makes sense, just like the world card in the major arcana or the dark moon preceding the new moon. The order of the runes is not arbitrary.

Dagaz nurtures a closeness with nature through consistency, routine, and ritual. Every morning we can trust that the sun won't sleep in and show up late. So how can we provide the same kind of devotional consistency within our practice and relationship to nature? Well, there's no easy answer to that, and admittedly, developing routines within my practice is something I have always struggled with. Many of us have kids, animals, relationships, and jobs that require much of our attention and energy.

I can't tell you how many times I've tried to have a meditation routine, a prayer routine, an offering routine, and I might do well for a week or three and eventually life happens and it fizzles out. Our lives are busy. There are two humans (including myself) and five animals in my house that require my attention and care. It's not an excuse, just a reality. My inability to keep a daily ritual going really did begin to weigh on me, however.

My solution to this consistency conundrum was to add spiritual aspects to some of the mundane tasks that need to be checked off daily, such as walking the dogs. Dog walking provides me with the opportunity to meditate and commune with the outdoors, even if only for a short while. I very much enjoy walking meditation, as sitting meditation tends to eventually result in back pain for me. Sure, there are interruptions, other people walking their dogs, poop stops (for my dogs, not me), loud cars . . . and just like in mindfulness meditation, I acknowledge the interruptions (and scoop the poop) and gently return to meditation. While small, this has been a revelation to me when it comes to routine. Rain or shine, the dogs need to be walked, which allows me to keep a consistent meditation routine.

Our daily "musts" vary from person to person. If you're a regular coffee or tea drinker, you may find that your morning cuppa provides an opportunity to leave an offering to your patron deity. You may even eventually get into the habit of pouring two cups instead of one. I have a miniature tea-cup that I've designated specifically to offerings. Some practitioners pair affirmations and mantras with their morning beverages, stirring in daily intentions and sipping mindfully. If you're often stuck in traffic during your morning commute, use the time to express gratitude for the blessings in your life, which ironically includes the car you're currently trapped in and the job you're on your way to. Meditate in the shower. Feel the water and suds on your skin, smell the scent of body washes and shampoo, hear the running water, see your naked body without judgment. Recite affirmations while brushing your teeth; not only will this put you in the right mindset, but the garbled speech is sure to elicit a chuckle. Perhaps when we begin to participate in these tiny routines, we inevitably hone the skill of consistency, which I believe is truly important for the serious practitioner of magick—especially one on the path to spiritual transformation.

It may be helpful to ask just as the sun shows up every morning: What can I show up for daily? In what ways can I be as reliable as the rising sun? As we get older, we realize that there just aren't enough hours in a day to accomplish everything we'd like, but as long as we're at least trying to maintain small routines in our practice, we are succeeding. I say small because these routines don't have to be anything elaborate. Life requires a list of small maintenance tasks we must perform daily to keep up on well-being, such as brushing our teeth, eating healthy meals, and getting some form of exercise. Keeping a car in good shape requires gas, air in the tires, oil changes, and tune-ups. Healthy relationships require honesty, communication, compromise, and intimacy. If your magickal practice is up there in priority alongside your relationships, hygiene, and health, then it may be useful to ask what small maintenance items can be performed daily to keep it in optimal condition. As witches, druids, pagans, et cetera, when we prioritize our magick and make it a part of daily life, we inevitably hold space for the natural world.

The best times to work with the Dagaz rune are during liminal times, such as sunrise and sunset as well as the equinoxes, as these times dwell in the balance of light and dark. The transformation rune is a reminder that change is the only constant. When it seems as though we can't fit anything more into our already packed schedules, the break-through rune shows up with the assist and teaches us how to make time for our magick. Dagaz is truly the driving force behind every change we seek to make for the better and wants to see us succeed in all we do.

The following is a ritual to support one as they undergo immense life changes.

What you'll need:

One black or white candle
One candleholder
Matches or a lighter
A bowl of water
An offering of your choice

The best time to perform the ritual is sunrise, sunset, or during the equinoxes.

Begin by choosing a quiet place where you will be undisturbed. Place the water and candle (I find that chime candles work best for this) directly in front of you within reach. Light the candle and state: *As Fire enters/exits* (enters for sunrise and Spring equinox and exits for sunset and Autumn equinox) *the sky, I call on the power of Dagaz, mighty rune of transformation, to aid me in my magick. With reverence and humility, I give you this offering of _____ .*

Pick up the candle, turn it on its side, and allow the wax to drip into the water while moving the candle in the shape of Dagaz and state: *As the wax transforms from liquid to solid with ease, I ask for the strength to accept and adapt to the changes in my life. Please aid me, Dagaz, as I navigate through unknown territory.*

Place the candle in its holder and keep your gaze fixed on the water and wax. Use this time to feel your heart and mind opening to the idea of change. Allow yourself time to reflect on gratitude for as long as you wish. Blow out the candle, gather and dispose of the wax drippings, and offer the water to the Earth. Hail, Dagaz and hail the runes!

CORRESPONDENCES OF DAGAZ

ELEMENT	Fire
ZODIAC	Pisces
PLANET	Sun, Pluto
MOON PHASE	All
TAROT	The World, Judgment
CRYSTAL	Rainbow Quartz
CHAKRA	Crown
DEITIES	Aurora, Cerridwen, Eos, Khepri, Nut, Nyx
PLANTS	Frankincense, Gum Mastic, Lobelia, Mandrake, Passionflower

The plants of Dagaz establish union of the physical and spiritual. Their powers are transformative, balancing, and elevating. In workings the following plants support tremendous growth of spirit.

Frankincense
(*Boswellia* spp.)

If you're familiar with the birth story of Jesus, you've likely heard of the three wise men who arrived bearing gifts, one of which was frankincense. This intensely purifying resin is a staple for prayer, ritual, and consecration as it raises vibrations and elevates consciousness. It is a mighty protector of the soul, spirit, and astral body. Frankincense is a key ally in exorcisms due to the ability to completely transform the energies within a space. I once heard a demonologist say, "If you want to repel a demon, burn frankincense. If you want to make a demon laugh, burn sage." Noted! Not to knock sage, as it can definitely work to transmute the energies of a space, but in a milder manner. This uplifting resin is ruled by the Sun and is appropriate for solar rituals, solstice celebrations, energy work, and spells for success. The incense aids in concentration during meditation and magick and is an excellent offering to deities. Paired with Dagaz, frankincense supports connection to all life and the cosmos as a whole.

Medicinal Properties

Frankincense is a staple in aromatherapy used to relieve stress, anxiety, and depression. It's seldom ingested these days but does have a history as an internal medicine, particularly within ayurveda. Traditionally, it served as a remedy for arthritis. It has been used to treat diarrhea, particularly that which results from Crohn's disease and ulcerative colitis. Folks with abdominal tumors or cystic fibrosis may benefit from the use of frankincense. It helps to bring on menstruation and soothe menstrual pain. The antiseptic properties make for a great topical medicine. Actions: analgesic, anti-inflammatory, antiseptic, astringent, carminative, emmenagogue, expectorant, nervine, sedative. Warming and drying. The essential oil may irritate sensitive skin. High doses may cause allergic reactions in some.

Gum Mastic
(*Pistacia lentiscus*)

Gum mastic is an aromatic tree resin found in the Mediterranean. It is best used for the raising of vibrations and banishing harmful energies.

Gum mastic is useful for those undergoing radical spiritual change and ascension, especially when combined with the Dagaz rune. Both the rune and resin promote a strong and smooth transformation. The resin is often burned during initiations, consecration, purification, and ceremonial magick.

Medicinal Properties

Traditional uses for gum mastic include treating coughs and bronchitis. Due to its antifungal properties, it is typically added to topical formulas for skin disorders, such as sores and boils. For centuries it has been used as a chewing gum to support dental health. Gum mastic remedies gastrointestinal upsets such as colitis, acid reflux, and Crohn's disease. It was used by the ancient Egyptians in the embalming process. Actions: antibacterial, antifungal, anti-inflammatory, antioxidant, antiseptic, digestive, hepatoprotective. Avoid during pregnancy and nursing.

Lobelia
(*Lobelia inflata*)

Lobelia promotes a state of overall well-being. It is protective of physical, mental, and spiritual health. It's ruled by the element of Water and the dreamy planet Neptune. The flowers encourage prophetic dreaming and aid in divination. This tropical plant encourages the release of what is no longer necessary and is therefore a wonderful plant to work with when purging toxic emotions and energies from the body. Traditionally, lobelia has been used to tame storms of extraordinary intensity and works equally as well at taming the emotional storms that rage within from time to time.

Medicinal Properties

Lobelia tincture provides relief for TMJ by relaxing the muscles that cause teeth grinding and clenching. Native Americans and Europeans used it to treat asthma and syphilis. Lobelia works on nicotine receptors (although it does not contain nicotine) and has been used to help people quit smoking. Due to its emetic properties, lobelia has also been known by the names pukeweed and gagroot. Actions: alterative, antispasmodic, diaphoretic, emetic, expectorant, nervine. Neutral and drying. Large doses can be toxic, resulting in drowsiness, vomiting, and respiratory failure. The fresh plant should never be ingested. Avoid while pregnant or breastfeeding.

Mandrake
(*Mandragora officinarum*)

Mandrake root is incredibly versatile and enjoys a long-held reputation as a powerfully magickal plant. Although it is often linked to baneful magick and death, it is a staunch protector from evil, especially demonic possession. Like most plants that yield intoxicating effects, some label mandrake as evil. Traditionally it is gathered ritually in the dark of night just before dawn on Fridays, due to its association with Venus. The mature mandrake root resembles a human body and has a long history of use as magickal poppets. It is ideal for communication with deities connected to death, such as Hel, Anubis, Sedna, or the Morrigan. The powdered root may be added to incense to help induce hypnotic states for otherworldly journeying. Mandrake also lends its powers to money, love, and sex magick. Those who are trying to conceive should place the root beneath their mattress. Folklore suggests the plant unleashes a ghastly scream when pulled from the ground—one that could possibly kill those within earshot. To avoid death but still obtain the root, it is said that the stems of mandrake were tied to the tails of dogs to uproot them. (Not cool, man.) Keep a piece of the root on an altar or mantle to invite joy and luck into the home and protect the inhabitants. Another traditional use is the carving of the root for talismans. Soak the root in water the night before Samhain, when the veil that separates us from the spirit world is at its thinnest. In the morning, with a finger or paint brush, use the water to trace the Dagaz rune on each door to block unwanted spirits while allowing in the invited.

Medicinal Properties

Mandrake is among the safer nightshades but should still be handled with extreme caution. Historically, its intoxicating effects were used as anesthesia preceding surgeries. Mandrake has an affinity for the liver, and in proper doses it can effectively support liver health. The leaves are cooling and have been used to relieve toothaches. Topically, it was used to relieve rheumatic pain, sunburn, and fever. Actions: analgesic, emetic, narcotic, nervine, purgative, soporific. Cold and drying. The root and bark are highly toxic in large doses. Consult a professional herbalist before working with mandrake.

Passionflower
(*Passiflora incarnata*)

As the name suggests, passionflower is associated with passion and love. A plant of Neptune and Venus, it makes the perfect offering for the goddesses Freyja and Frigga (who are sometimes thought to be one and the same), Aphrodite, and Hathor. Passionflower isn't solely associated with *romantic* love, but also self, friend, and familial love. Carry in a yellow sachet to attract new friendships. Passionflower helps to ease mood swings, anger, and intense sadness. I've chosen Dagaz as the rune of passionflower due to its affinity for balance, wellness, and personal transformation. It helps one to recenter, promotes tranquility, quiets mental chatter, and fosters relaxation and focus. Use as an incense when emotional balance is needed. Passionflower is a wonderful additive to home-blessing incense blends as it encourages peace among the inhabitants of the home.

Medicinal Properties
Passionflower is a great ally for those who are high strung or restless. It soothes the central nervous system and lowers blood pressure. It is perfect for those who suffer from insomnia because not only does it help one fall asleep, it also helps them stay asleep. Passionflower may be used to ease spasms, hiccups, tremors, convulsions, and tension. Its sedative effects are comparable to those of valerian root. Taken as an infusion or tincture, passionflower helps to ease the overactive mind. Actions: analgesic, antibacterial, antidepressant, antifungal, anti-inflammatory, antispasmodic, aphrodisiac, diaphoretic, hypotensive, nervine, sedative. Cooling and drying. May cause drowsiness. Avoid large doses during pregnancy and nursing. The unripe fruit is toxic.

CONCLUSION

I hope that you have found worthwhile information within these pages—information that can help you elevate your own personal craft and empower you as a witch. When we find our niche among the many branches of witchcraft, we gain a sense of personal power and satisfaction. My practice started out largely eclectic and while it still is for the most part, it really began to take shape when I discovered my love for plant medicine, ritual, and lore. Only a short time after the start of my plant explorations I was introduced to the runes, and that's what really sealed my identity as a *witch*.

Whether you call yourself a heathen, witch, pagan, shaman, occultist, mystic, or you don't call yourself anything at all, I think the one thing we can all agree on is that we're searching for more beyond what many accept as whole reality. Not only do we want answers to life's big mysteries, but we actively work to obtain the knowledge we seek, and we do so with the help of allies like runes, plants, tarot, crystals, meditation, and more. We are alchemists and seekers of progress and truth. We flourish in the dissection of what we're told is real (or *not* real). Regardless of our titles or lack thereof, we are fully aware that we are not just earthly bodies, we are cosmic spirits, too. What exactly does that mean? Well, that's precisely what we're all trying to find out.

I wish you endless growth, love, wisdom, and magick on your journey.

APPENDIX

THE RUNIC FORMULARY

Now the fun begins! As a witch is there anything more rewarding than creating potions, incense, remedies, and spell jars? Personally, I don't think so. In the following paragraphs I have included some of my time-tested blends for you to try and modify. The information in this book may be used to arm you with the knowledge you need to create your very own herbal formulas safely and effectively. Always make sure the plant matter chosen is safe for your purpose whether it be for consumption, skin application, or fumigation. When you're sure the plants you've chosen are safe for your creation, go wild! Experiment! I can't tell you how many horrible tasting teas I've drunk from a tea blend that I thought was a good idea. That's how you learn, though—through trial and error. With practice you'll learn which herbs complement each other in a variety of ways. I highly recommend keeping a notebook and recording all of your formulations and impressions. Before we move on to the runic formulas, let's take a look at the various methods at your disposal.

Incense Blends

Loose incense is fun and easy to make. The first step is selecting your dried plants and resins. Having a mortar and pestle is helpful. Coffee grinders are ideal for the tougher parts of plants such as the roots. Finely powdered incense will produce a lot of smoke and quickly burn through. Larger pieces of dried plant material and resins provide a slower burn. Once you've ground your desired herbs and resins, simply mix them together and store in a jar away from direct sunlight. Loose incense burns best on charcoal, which should be placed in either a heat-safe dish or cauldron. Incense is often used in ritual for purposes of purification and consecration and to shift one's consciousness, but you can make an incense for any purpose. It also makes for a fantastic offering.

Tinctures

When making tinctures the first step is choosing your herbs and menstruum. The menstruum is the liquid that will extract the medicinal constituents from the plant material. Alcohol, glycerin, and vinegar are the most common choices for menstruum. Alcohol tends to work best for extractions (except for mucilaginous herbs, which macerate best in glycerin), but it may not be the best choice for children or people who choose to avoid alcohol. In-depth instructions on tincture-making are beyond the scope of this book; if it's something that you're interested in learning, I recommend picking up a book on herbal medicine making. Tinctures can have a shelf life of up to three years if stored properly out of the light in a temperature-controlled environment. This type of herbal remedy is best used as preventative medicine.

Infused Oils

The process for making infused oils is very similar to tincture preparation. First, you'll choose your herbs (always dry), essential oils, and carrier oil (e.g., olive, grapeseed, jojoba). As with any preparation I like to communicate to the plants their role in the blend and offer gratitude during the process. The maceration process for infused oils can be accomplished in a variety of ways. One way is to store it in a dark space for six weeks, remembering to shake it regularly. Using a double boiler is a much faster method, and the infused oil can be completed in roughly three to four hours. Solar infusions use the power and warmth of the sun for the maceration process; simply leave the jar in a sunny spot for three weeks and remember to shake it daily. Vitamin E oil may be added to the mixture as a preservative. Infused oils have a shelf life of one to two years. Jojoba oil is my preferred carrier oil as it has a longer shelf life than most carriers. Infused oils are ideal for blessings (of both people as well as ritual items), drawing magickal symbols on the body, anointing chakras, and as additions to ritual baths.

Teas

We all know teas. You steep it, you drink it. Boom, done. A typical tea steeps for five to ten minutes while a medicinal tea steeps overnight in an enclosed teapot. In the morning the plant material is strained and the tea may be refrigerated and used for up to three days. Drinking tea prior to a ritual is one way to invoke the desired energies needed to achieve your goal. Teas are also excellent for offerings.

Sprays

To make an herbal spray, the first step is to steep the dried plant matter in hot water just as you would tea. I love to use moon, rain, and snow water, but any water you have will do fine. The longer you leave the plant matter to steep, the more the spirit of the plants and medicinal constituents will be extracted into the water. Once the tea has cooled, add about one part vodka (as a preservative) to five parts tea. Bottle and add your favorite essential oils. Herbal sprays are often used as incense alternatives for small spaces and folks who have an intolerance to smoke.

Bath Blends

When making bath blends, select herbs and essential oils are mixed with Epsom salts and a bit of baking soda (optional). If having loose herbs in your tub is a no-go due to drainage issues, first prepare a large pot of tea from the herbs selected. Strain out the plant matter and add to your bathwater with essential oils and a cup of Epsom salts. Large tea balls are great for this, too. Bath blends are used to cleanse and imbue the witch with certain energies typically pre-ritual. Post-ritual bath blends are best after magickal workings that may have attracted undesirable energies.

Spell Bottles

Spell bottles and sachets are perfect for when you want to make an herbal preparation but not necessarily one to burn, ingest, or apply to the skin. All you need is a small glass jar with a lid or cork followed by your dried plant material. Depending on what the spell bottle is for, other common items to add are crystal chips, sigils, hair, fingernails, drops of blood, seashells, and sand. Once complete, spell bottles serve as energetic charms that advocate for the practitioner's intentions.

The following blends include some of my own as well as general suggestions. They are not set in stone and may be modified to best suit your needs.

FEHU

❧ Money Maker Ritual Oil ☙

Alfalfa
Basil
Cinquefoil
Chamomile
Cedar essential oil
Pine essential oil
Sunflower oil

❧ Success Spell Bottle ☙

Green aventurine chips
Bay leaves
Allspice
Peppermint
Rose hips
Sunflower seeds
Calendula
Chicory

URUZ ᚢ

❧ Vital Energy Tea ☙

Echinacea root
Elderberries
Green tea
Cinnamon
Nutmeg

THURISAZ ᚦ

❧ Shield Me Spritz ☙

Nettle
Hyssop
Angelica
Dill seeds
Agrimony
Frankincense essential oil
Lavender essential oil

ANSUZ ᚨ

❧ Clear Communication Incense ☙

Sage
Clove
Anise
Uva ursi
Cedar bark

❧ Truth Seeker Divination Oil ☙

Yarrow
Thyme
Mugwort
Eyebright
Vervain

Spikenard essential oil
Clary sage essential oil
Grapeseed oil

RAIDHO ᚱ

❧ In Control Spell Jar ❧

Ginger
Calamus
Basil
Yarrow
Thyme
Comfrey
Solomon's seal
Obsidian chips

KENAZ ᚲ

❧ Creative Fire Tea ❧

Rose hips
Ginger
Cinnamon
Cardamom
Clove
Vervain

❧ Love and Lust Oil ❧

Damiana
Rose
Jasmine
Shatavari
Saw palmetto
Rose quartz chips
Ylang-ylang essential oil
Olive oil

GEBO X

❧ In Balance Tincture ❧

Tulsi
Ashwagandha
Astragalus
Licorice Root
Reishi

WUNJO ᚹ

❧ Good Vibrations Oil ❧

Anise
Lemon balm
Lavender
Marshmallow root
Rose
Honeysuckle
Sunflower oil

❧ Grief Relief Tea (or bath) ❧

Hawthorn berries
White willow bark
Sarsaparilla
Marjoram
Red clover
Honey

HAGALAZ ᚺ

❧ Bad Bitch Oil ❧

Dragon's blood resin
Rose
Clove
Nettle

Bay leaves
Mugwort
Dong quai
Myrrh essential oil
Rose essential oil
Jojoba oil

NAUTHIZ ✝

∽ Emotional Healing Tincture ∽

Lemon balm
Motherwort
Ashwagandha
Chamomile
Skullcap

ISA |

∽ Baby, It's Cold Outside Tea ∽

Ginger
Cardamom
Clove
Cinnamon
Dandelion root
Vanilla bean
Red rooibos

∽ Be Still Tea

(May cause drowsiness. Avoid before operating a motor vehicle.)

Kava kava
Chamomile
Lemon balm
Passionflower
Cinnamon
Honey

JERA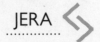

❧ Smooth Transition Tincture ❧

> Dong quai
> Lavender
> Clove
> Tulsi
> Skullcap

EIHWAZ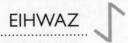

❧ You Are Remembered Incense ❧
(an offering to the dead)

> Calendula
> Rosemary
> Dittany of Crete
> Anise
> Myrrh

PERTHRO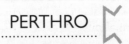

❧ Cosmic Consciousness Spell Bottle ❧

> Uva ursi
> Rue
> Sage
> Anise
> Goldenrod
> Tulsi
> Gotu kola
> White willow bark
> Labradorite chips

❧ Fertility Oil ❧

Flax Seed
Lady's mantle
Raspberry leaf
Motherwort
Blessed thistle
Shatavari
Ylang-ylang essential oil
Grapeseed oil

ELHAZ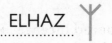

❧ Divine Protection Spritz ❧

Bay
Basil
Mullein
Lavender
Angelica
Hyssop
Juniper berries
Sandalwood essential oil

SOWILO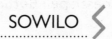

❧ Solar Energy Oil ❧

Calendula
Sunflower
Dandelion
Eyebright
Frankincense essential oil
Safflower oil
Citrine chips

TEIWAZ ↑

❧ Courage Tea ☙

Borage
Ginger
Turmeric
Galangal
Lemon

BERKANA ᛒ

❧ Rebirth Bath ☙

Spearmint
Calendula
Violet
Passionflower
Epsom salts
Baking soda
Bergamot essential oil

❧ A Mother's Love Tincture ☙

Motherwort
Milky oats
Chamomile
Catnip
Tulsi

EHWAZ ᛖ

❧ Animal Protection Spell Jar ☙

Dill
Cedar
Basil
Catnip

Mullein
Angelica
Red clover
Maple leaf or bark
Fur from the animal (a few pieces of shed fur; no need to give your
pet a haircut)

MANNAZ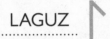

❧ Brain Potion Tincture ❧

Ginkgo
Gotu kola
Reishi
Ashwagandha
Butterfly pea blossom

LAGUZ

❧ Lunar Energy Oil ❧

Jasmine
Bladderwrack
Mugwort
Lotus
Violet
Camphor essential oil
Lavender essential oil

INGWAZ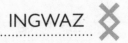

❧ Unlock Potential Tea ❧

Fenugreek
Lavender
Lemongrass
Hibiscus
Rose hips

OTHALA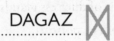

❧ Protect My Home Spritz or Floor Cleanser Additive ☙

Avens

Angelica

Blackberry leaves

Meadowsweet

Witch hazel

Moon water

Eucalyptus essential oil

Add some blackberry thorns to the final formula

DAGAZ

❧ Awaken the Spirit Tea ☙

Black tea

Passionfruit

Hibiscus

Orange peel

Rose hips

Licorice root

Eleuthero

Lemon

GLOSSARY

Abortifacient—Brings on abortion

Adaptogen—Aids the body in adapting to stressors and promotes the normalizing of bodily processes

Adrenal—Refers to a pair of ductless glands above the kidneys

Alexiteric—Resists venom or poison

Alterative—Purifies the blood

Analgesic—Pain reliever

Antacid—Neutralizes stomach acidity

Antibacterial—Fights against and prevents bacterial growth

Antiedemic—Reduces edema

Antiemetic—Relieves nausea and vomiting

Antifungal—Fights against and prevents fungal growth

Antihistamine—Compounds used to treat allergies

Antioxidant—Inhibits damaging oxidation

Antiplatelet—Inhibits platelet aggregation to maintain healthy arterial circulation

Antipyretic—Prevents or reduces fever

Antiseptic—Prevents the growth of harmful microorganisms

Antispasmodic—Relieves muscle spasms

Antivenomous—Opposes the action of venom

Antiviral—Fights and prevents viruses

Anxiolytic—Reduces anxiety

Aquaretic—Promotes increased urination without the loss of electrolytes

Aromatic—Plants that emit pleasant scents

Astringent—Contracts skin cells and bodily tissue

Bitter—Plant extracts that stimulate the production of bile in the liver, which in turn improves digestion and absorption

Bronchodilator—Causes opening of the bronchioles

Carminative—Relieves flatulence

Cathartic—Accelerates bowel evacuation

Cholagogue—Stimulates gallbladder contractions to secrete bile

Choleretic—Stimulates bile production from the liver

Cicatrizant—Builds scar tissue in the process of healing wounds

Circulatory—Relates to the movement of blood

Decongestant—Relieves nasal congestion

Demulcent—An oily substance that soothes inflammation of the mucous membranes

Detoxifier—Removes harmful substances

Diaphoretic—Induces perspiration

Digestive—Promotes proper food digestion

Diuretic—Promotes increased urination

Emetic—Triggers vomiting

Emmenagogue—Stimulates menstrual flow

Emollient—Moisturizes

Estrogenic—Regulator of female hormones

Expectorant—Treats coughs by promoting secretion of sputum within air passages

Febrifuge—Prevents or reduces fever

Galactagogue—Stimulates the production of breast milk

Hemostatic—Compresses vessels to stop the flow of blood

Hepatoprotective—Prevents liver damage

Hypotensive—Low blood pressure

Laxative—Stimulates bowel evacuation

Mucilaginous—A viscous consistency

Narcotic—Eases severe pain, induces sleep, and alters mood

Nervine—Calms the nerves

Neuroprotective—Supports proper functioning of the nervous system

Nootropic—Enhances memory and cognitive function

Nutritive—Nourishing

Oxytocic—Hastens childbirth

Parturient—A person or animal about to give birth

Poultice—Mass of moist plant material applied to the skin to relieve inflammation or soreness

Purgative—Strongly laxative

Refrigerant—Promotes cooling

Restorative—Having the ability to restore balance, strength, and health

Rubefacient—Increases redness in the skin by increasing circulation

Sedative—Induces calmness and sleep

Sialagogue—Encourages production of saliva

Soporific—Causes drowsiness and induces sleep

Sternutatory—Induces sneezing

Stimulant—Any substance used to excite a bodily function

Stomachic—Promotes appetite and healthy digestion

Tonic—Any substance that provides invigoration and a sense of well-being

Vasodilator—Dilates the blood vessels

Vermifuge—Expels parasitic worms

Vulnerary—Heals wounds

BIBLIOGRAPHY

Apelian, Nicole and Claude Davis. *The Lost Book of Herbal Remedies*. N.p.: Global Brother, 2021.

Aswynn, Freya. *Northern Mysteries and Magick*. St. Paul, Minn.: Llewellyn Worldwide, 1998.

Beyerl, Paul. *The Master Book of Herbalism*. Custer, Wash.: Phoenix Publishing Co., 1984.

Brewer, Gregory Michael. *The Ancient Magick of Trees*. Woodbury, Minn.: Llewellyn Worldwide, 2019.

Butterworth, Lisa. *The Beginner's Guide to Crystals: The Everyday Magic of Crystal Healing, with 65+ Stones*. New York: Ten Speed Press, 2019.

Chevallier, Andrew. *Encyclopedia of Herbal Medicine*. London, England: Penguin Random House, 2016.

Cohen, Deatra and Adam Siegel. *Ashkenazi Herbalism: Rediscovering the Herbal Traditions of Eastern European Jews*. Berkeley, Calif.: North Atlantic Books, 2021.

Crowley, Aleister. *Magick, Liber ABA, Book 4*. York Beach, Maine: Weiser Books, 1994.

Easley, Thomas and Steven Horne. *The Modern Herbal Dispensatory: A Medicine-Making Guide*. Berkeley, Calif.: North Atlantic Books, 2016.

Greer, John Michael. *Encyclopedia of Natural Magic*. St. Paul, Minn.: Llewellyn, 2019.

Grieve, Maud. "Aconite." Botanical.com (website), 2021.

———. "Avens." Botanical.com (website), 2021.

———. "Blackberry." Botanical.com (website), 2021.

Harrison, Karen. *The Herbal Alchemist's Handbook: A Complete Guide to Magickal Herbs and How to Use Them*. Newburyport, Mass.: Weiser Books, 2020.

Hopman, Ellen Evert. *The Sacred Herbs of Samhain: Plants to Contact the Spirits of the Dead*. Rochester, Vt.: Destiny Books, 2019.

Lee, Min-sun, Juyoung Lee, Bum-Jin Park, and Yoshifumi Miyazaki. "Interaction with Indoor Plants May Reduce Psychological and Physiological Stress by Suppressing Autonomic Nervous System Activity in Young Adults: A Randomized Crossover Study." *Journal of Physiological Anthropology* 34, no. 1 (2015): 21.

Levine, Noah. *Dharma Punx: A Memoir*. San Francisco: HarperCollins, 2003.

Lindrooth, Charis. "When in Doubt, Try Nettles!" BotanicWise (website), 2023.

Loðursson, Ljóssál. *Ginnrúnbók*. N.p.: Fall of Man, 2021.

Mars, Brigitte and Chrystle Fiedler. *The Home Reference to Holistic Health and Healing*. Beverly, Mass.: Fair Winds Press, 2015.

McCarthy, Juliana. *The Stars Within You: A Modern Guide to Astrology*. Boulder, Colo.: Roost Books, 2018.

Michael, Coby. *The Poison Path Herbal: Baneful Herbs, Medicinal Nightshades, and Ritual Entheogens*. Rochester, Vt.: Park Street Press, 2021.

Neves, Liz. *Northeast Medicinal Plants: Identify, Harvest, and Use 111 Wild Herbs for Health and Wellness*. Portland, Ore.: Timber Press, 2020.

Paine, Angela. *Healing Plants of the Celtic Druids*. Winchester, UK: Moon Books, 2017.

Patterson, Rachel. *Curative Magic: A Witch's Guide to Self-Discovery, Care & Healing*. Woodbury, Minn.: Llewellyn Publications, 2020.

Paxson, Diana. *Taking Up the Runes: A Complete Guide to Using Runes in Spells, Rituals, Divination, and Magic*. Boston, Mass.: Red Wheel/Weiser LLC, 2005.

Penczak, Christopher. *The Inner Temple of Witchcraft: Magick, Meditation, and Psychic Development*. Woodbury, Minn.: Llewellyn Publications, 2003.

Pollack, Rachel. *Seventy-Eight Degrees of Wisdom*. Wellingborough, England: Aquarian Press, 1980.

Robbins, Jim. "How Immersing Yourself in Nature Benefits Your Health." *PBS News Hour* (website), January 13, 2020.

Sheffield, Ann Gróa. *Long Branches: Runes of the Younger Futhark*. Self-published, Lulu.com, 2013.

Shoemaker, SaVanna. "All You Need to Know about Figs." *Healthline* (website), June 3, 2020.

Steward, Amy. *Wicked Plants: The Weed that Killed Lincoln's Mother & Other Botanical Atrocities.* Chapel Hill, N.C.: Algonquin Books of Chapel Hill, 2009.

Tierra, Michael. *Planetary Herbology: An Integration of Western Herbs into the Traditional Chinese and Ayurvedic Systems.* Twin Lakes, Wisc.: Lotus Press, 1988.

Winston, David and Steven Maimes. *Adaptogens: Herbs for Strength, Stamina, and Stress Relief.* Rochester, Vt.: Healing Arts Press, 2007.

INDEX